THE GLUCOSE RUSE BLUES

THE RUSE THAT GLUES
YOUR BLUES TO THEIR DUES
(without the color)

Copyright 2018

ISBN: 9781987436587

Forward

This short synopsis of the devastation that the chemical industry is imposing on the American people and the world is an abbreviated tale of the most devastating practice to ever hit mankind.

I'm publishing this smaller evidence of what they're doing so that I can tell as many people as possible of the danger in consuming their glyphosate soaked grains.

After losing 3 family members to the ravages of cancer, 3 members to heart disease, and then more to Alzheimer's disease, I've come to the conclusion that this must come to an end. It's time that this scourge continued no more. The sooner it can happen isn't soon enough.

The scourge I speak of is the Glucose Ruse. It's a designed trap to force your need for medications. But, what if there is a way out of this scourge? The way out, unfortunately is only known to a few who have taken the time to learn about it.

Now's your chance. If you ever wondered why your head hurts or why you wake up in pain, read on and learn. Learn what you can do about it and DO IT! This is life saving at its simplest. It's just not the easiest.

Because of the number of technical terms in this book that are hard to understand, I suggest just skimming over the PubMed entries that have many of these hard to read terms. I included them simply to prove my argument and not to confuse anyone. Any reference to Monsanto is to Monsanto and not the new owner of Monsanto, Bayer.

The information you'll find in this volume will amaze you about what you don't know, about what you're eating. If you choose to follow my advice, your ultimate savings in medications alone will astound you. You'll be removing most all medicines from your shopping lists. Your savings in food that's harms you will be your greatest asset.

DO YOU EVER FEEL, "out of sorts"?
IT'S THIS GLUCOSE RUSE
THAT'S AT THE BASE OF ALL THE PAIN
FOR THE DRUGS YOU USE

Table of Contents

1) VICTIMIZED, WE'VE BEEN Crimes of the Food Industry;   04
2) CALORIES, CARBS, AND THEIR LURE   10
3) THE CELEBRATION OF ADDICTION   24
   Why the food industry wants you to feed your addiction
4) THE DANGERS OF GLYCATION   53
5) ADDING THE CHEMICALS THAT ALTER YOUR HEALTH   100
   The Glyphosate Poisoning of America
6) THE REAL REASON TERRORISM EXISTS and THRIVES   114
7) FDA and THEIR TAKE ON GLUTEN   124
8) USDA's Propensity to cover-up the tainting of the grains   140
   to sell more for the farmer and influence the FDA
9) THE RESTAURANT RUSE OF THE GLUCOSE BLUES   157
10) THE POWER OF FASTING   165
11) THE BENEFIT OF FAT, YOUR POWER FOOD   182
12) THE BLISS OF KETOSIS   197
    MY PLEA TO THEE   208

THERE IS A PRICE AS YOU WILL SEE

TO FEED YOUR ADDICTION GLEEFULLY

IT BRINGS ALL DEATH PREMATURELY

ALL WHILE LIVING LIFE PAINFULLY

I
VICTIMIZED, WE'VE BEEN

Crimes of the Food Industry

MISLED WE'VE BEEN, ALL OF THESE YEARS
TO EAT THEIR FOOD TO DRIVE OUR TEARS.

Do you ever get headaches? I used to. I used to get them quite often. But then I used to eat a lot more carbs, than what I do now. I've learned a hell of a lot since I gave up all the carbs. I learned that what you and I have been told for over 50 years is exactly the opposite of what we should have been told, in respects as to what to eat. We've been lied to. And corporations are wreaking profits from this ruse. We've been subjected to a ruse so grandiose, it dwarves all ruses before it.

This ruse minimizes any addiction, terror, death tolls from catastrophes, even death tolls from any disease or deaths from all wars, that have ever existed, as this ruse is responsible for the equivalency of all deaths from all modern diseases and addictions. This myth has killed far more people than any other single reason. Right now, it's killing people at a toll of 123,287 people every day. That would wipe out 100 towns like what I grew up in, in one day. How long would it take to wipe out your city?

There's only one reason for this myth to exist, and that's to feed the greed of the investors in the industries that are perpetuating this myth. The myth? You need carbs and you need them, in abundance. The biggest myth? The more sweets you eat, the more fun life is. You see this in all the advertising for sodas, candy, and snacks. The reality? The more sweets you eat, the sooner you'll suffer the consequences. All addictions have consequences. (That's why they don't want you to know what they do, in their perpetuation of this ruse.)

Welcome to the **GLUCOSE RUSE**

THE RUSE OF YOUR LIFETIME

Enjoy life to the fullest extent that you can, with all the carbs you want to eat and drink, but don't worry about your health. We've got that covered, with treatment, drugs, and therapy all designed to ease the pain and life threatening conditions that our food will eventually give you. We've got hospitals, nursing homes, and clinics all lined up waiting to admit you, for your cancer, heart disease, or Alzheimer's disease. We promise you you'll enjoy the trip, until you get sick. Yet, we've got all the meds you'll need to quell your aches and pains. If you get addicted to any of those, we've got therapy sessions to break that addiction. If you have any side effects from our medications, we got other medications to ease that discomfort, so have another corn chip, or potato chip with your hot dog or hamburger, and cola or beer, and let us entertain you, while you sit back and get sick, for us to treat. (This is the ultimate trick or treat. Your treats, turned into their tricks.)

Our nation of capitalism, has designed an entire way of enjoying life, without regard to any kind of health consequences, either physical, financial, or spiritual. Well, on second thought, there might be some spiritual influence with this ruse. It does have a way of bringing families together...but that's after it tears them apart.

What they don't have, nor would they probably share it with you, if they did, is a way to break their initial addiction, the one to glucose. This is an addiction that all are born into and live with throughout the entirety of our lives. It's also an addiction, they use against us to their advantage.

If, we're to break this curse of addiction, we must end the use of the perpetuating cause of the myth. But, what is the cause of this myth? The entire cause of this myth is quite possibly, your favorite food. A Coke and a hot dog, or hamburger with your chips and beer, the all American favorites.

All of this food, gets glyphosated, multiple times before harvest. That something we'll be talking more about in Chapter 5. But it has magnified the dangers of these mostly grain foods, along with a host of vegetables (potatoes mostly).

What's needed to lose this ruse is to stop the perpetuation of it. The chemical/crop seed/food industry must cease and desist in their industrial farming, the designing of our disease and death, by spraying chemicals, forcing farmers, denying the danger, killing bees, and false advertising their benefits.

1. Growing food that shuts down the ability to perceive the damage it creates, as it's being done, to keep people fully duped to their ruse, the Glucose Ruse. Their carbs are engineered to dull your senses, so you don't notice what they're doing to you. They do it with their glyphosate pesticide. But then, this is the nature of sugar also. This is its addictive nature. This is why sugar is addictive and why it should be considered a drug, and regulated as so. The chemicals being dumped on these crops multiple times throughout their life cycle, are designed to keep you hungry by inhibiting enzymatic action in your body that tells you when to stop eating (you don't feel satiated as easily anymore), so you eat more and more. This is a never-ending cycle, that only worsens, the more you eat.

2. Spraying of enzyme-inhibiting chemicals on our food crops and our feed crops with the intention of selling more and more glyphosate. Now, farmers are spaying glyphosate to the tune of a million gallons a year on our food. This does multiple things to damage our bodies. The chemicals that kill the weeds in the field, are slowly, ever so slowly, taking our health. How quick you lose your health depends on how much sugar and starch you eat. The more you eat, the quicker your demise. These chemicals not only slow down your rate of satiation, they inhibit your ability to fully digest what you eat, increasing your hunger, to make you eat more and more and more. These chemicals also inhibit your sleep. Have you been having trouble sleeping lately?

3. Forcing farmers to plant. grow, and spray their crops with glyphosate *Roundup*, through the use of their GMO seeds. Monsanto, now owned by Bayer, owns 15 seed companies all selling GMO seed to feed your need to eat glyphosated crops. Because their glyphosate increases the addictive factor, it makes it even that more deadly. Because it inhibits proper digestion, it makes you eat more. Because it inhibits your sleep, it makes you eat when you're supposed to sleep. Monsanto knows this and they're spreading it as wide as they can, just to sell more Roundup.

4. Denying the damage and insisting that their glyphosate pesticide is safe and beneficial for mankind, when all it does is kill the environment, poison the groundwater, drastically damage bee populations, and lastly but not least, create your senescence. This is the real danger of this pesticide. By inhibiting enzymatic action in your body, these chemicals produce the same senescence in you, that they produce in weeds to kill them. Instead of killing you in 3 days, it takes anywhere from months to years, since your ingestion of the chemicals is so minute, each time you take it in. But, because it's sprayed on virtually every grain, you eat it all the time if you're

eating comfort foods, snack foods, and soda pop. All food designed to keep you addicted and wanting more to satisfy your hunger.

5. Killing off bee populations with their spraying. Since the mid-2000's many bees have been affected by *Colony Collapse Disorder*, which has had a disastrous effect on bee populations. The runoff taints about 40% the groundwater with their enzyme inhibiting chemicals, Chemicals proven to cause cancer, heart disease, Alzheimer's disease, all other dementias, and all other diseases of inflammation. All you have to do is look at the graphs of the increase of these diseases. They mirror the increase of glyphosate spraying, and yet, it criminally continues. According to *Bee Culture;*

"Pollinator Habitat Is Disappearing At Rates Usually Reserved For Descriptions Of Amazon Rain Deforestation"
"Glyphosate was detected in more than 50 percent of soil and sediment samples, and water samples from ditches and drains, precipitation, large rivers, and streams. Glyphosate was detected in less than 40 percent of water samples from lakes, ponds, wetlands. AMPA was detected in more than 80 percent of wastewater treatment plant samples, while glyphosate was detected in about 10 percent of those samples."

6. Recommendations to eat more grains and their tainted food, and to not eat what's really healthy. Why does the USDA and the FDA recommend what we eat, be more of the tainted food grown by all industrial farming? It's because they want you to eat what they can produce the most of. It's a matter of profit, and not necessarily health. This is a practice that must stop if our society is to ever get healthy.

All recommendations of diet must be based on what's healthy for the body and not what's healthy for the industry, such as ;

1. Fat is healthy to eat. In all reality, fat is the healthiest high octane food you can put in your body. Fat is more than twice as nutritious, as far as energy is concerned than glucose.

2. Carbohydrates initiate the process of glycation which is at the root of all disease. Without glucose, glycation can't take place. With glycation being at the root of all disease, if remove the glucose, you remove the glycation and thus, the disease. Without glycation taking place in the body, the body can't get sick. It automatically stays healthy.

3. Dispel the myth that high cholesterol is bad. High cholesterol is where your energy comes from, not glucose. Glucose makes cholesterol, but the wrong kind. The kind of cholesterol you get from carbs and glucose is a

dirty cholesterol. That is the foundation of Apo B LDL particles, which hold the foundation of more disease than any other type of LDL particle (there's 6 types of cholesterol particles, all designated by its core lipoprotein, the apolipoprotein). Apolipoprotein B is at the root of most disease because it's generated by, more than anything, carbs. Carbs make the dirtiest fuel for your body. That's why it creates so much disease.

4. MILK IS GOOD all milk fats are MCTs, the healthiest saturated fat you can eat. It's well established that MCTs are good for the body. What has yet to be established is how good milk fats are for the body. All milk fats are MCTs. That makes them the healthiest fats the body can ingest. That makes cream and butter healthy, much healthier than creamer and oleo. Those are recipes for disease. Creamer is all sugar and little more. Oleo is all vegetable oil, which can contribute to cancer, because of its omega 6 oils. All vegetable oils are long chain triglycerides (LCTs), instead of MCTs like those of butter & cream, Coconut oil, Palm Kernel oil, and Avocado oil

This is the basis of the Glucose Ruse, the worst scourge to ever hit mankind. In all reality, we were born into it, but we have a chemical industry that has a lot of money invested in pharmaceuticals and they've found out how they can affect our health, to need their pharmaceuticals by making their food more glycative than it's ever been.

So, who's guilty of perpetuating this Glucose Ruse? A chemical industry, bent on earning profits for their shareholders. A chemical industry, that owns at least 15 crop seed companies, all selling GMO seed that's Roundup ready. That means that it can absorb Roundup, which kills weeds through an action called senescence. Senescence is the science of aging and Roundup kills weeds by making them age super fast. So fast that they die in 3 days.

What happens when you ingest this glyphosate? What does it do to your body? Glyphosate inhibits enzymes. This is how it kills weeds. This is also what it does to your body. It just takes your body longer to die, because you eat little bits at a time when you take it in.

The enzymes it affects, affect your digestion, hunger, and sleep. If you have any problems in any of these areas, this is why. You're eating your problems when you eat carbs. So why would these carbs be at the root of all disease? In one word, glycation. What is this glycation?

Glycation is what creates AGEs, Advanced Glycation Endproducts. Every doctor knows about these nasty little buggers. They keep finding more and more of them each day. What they're not looking at when they research glycation to find medicines to counteract its disease-causing properties, is what would happen if they just removed the catalyzing agent. The catalyzing agent? Glucose. And, glucose comes from all carbs and sugar. Without glucose, glycation can't take place, making glucose the bad player in this play.

If products with glucose create a need for more medication, in order to sell more drugs, it would help enormously to sell more products that create that need. Fortunately for them, those products that they need to sell, are already addictive, making it that much easier to sell them. This is the celebration of our addiction and it's done on a societal level. This is evidence of the power of addiction, especially when it's legal.

Since this addiction is a legal addiction, it can be promoted without consequence, except to the ones who buy into it. They pay the deepest price for this addiction with their obesity, diabetes, arthritis, CVDs, cancer, lupus, fibromyalgia, Alzheimer's disease, Parkinson's disease, Pick's disease, the list is endless of all the diseases that carbs are at the root of.

Is it any wonder that this industry would want to keep this, quiet? How much would it cut into their profits if people knew about this ruse? Who would be left to buy their pharmaceuticals? Is this why they still perpetuate this ruse?

All they have to do is supply the seed to feed it and with 15 crop seed companies, they're set up to do exactly that, so they do. They do so legally, too. That is something we should be ashamed of. It's obviously a "feed our addiction" ploy to keep us addicted and to need their medicine, In the future.

If you can recommend your foods, you know will force the need for your medications, you're going to do so. If you can control the agency that makes these recommendations, you can control what they recommend, which is exactly what happens in our USDA and FDA. This industry also has reps working in the EPA and probably the CDC as well. Their influence is insurmountable in this industry. The only way to beat it is to not buy into it. But then the way I figure, who would, if they knew better?

II
CALORIES, DO YOU WORRY ABOUT THEM?

Calories, do you worry about how many you eat? If you do, you're not alone. A lot of people do the very same thing, they count their calories. If you're one of those who do, I have a suggestion for you. To help make your job easier and you healthier; it's not how many calories you eat, that's important. What's important is where the calories come from.

Calories are essential to survive, so they're absolutely necessary and yes if you eat more, you might weigh more. If you eat less, though, you don't always weigh less. That only applies, if you're eating carbs. You can't lose weight by eating less fat (but you can if you eat too much), as that's part of the ruse. That does make eating fewer calories crucial if you're eating carbs, yet eating less to control them can be very difficult, especially, if you're on a carb diet. The simple reason for this is because carbs make you hungry. They create and maintain a hunger cycle that you have no control over, without removing them. That makes, where you get your calories from, more important than how many you eat. In *It's Time for a Cure*, I show you how to eat more calories and lose weight.

Are the calories you get from the food you eat most, from carbohydrates or are they calories, from protein and fat? If you're eating calories from carbohydrates, under the guise of *healthy energy*, you're allowing those carbs to make the fat that your body needs to use for that energy. If you're getting your calories from fat and protein, you're feeding your body exactly what it needs to survive, thrive, and heal, better than you could ever imagine. Eating fats and protein also allows your body to heal itself from virtually anything, because glycation isn't involved, in a ketogenic diet. There is very little our bodies cannot heal from, as long as we don't have the influence of the glycation, that's the result of carbohydrates contaminating our systems. That means if your body needs glucose, let it make its own.

Whatever glucose you can get from carbs, your body can supply, on its own. When, certain parts of your brain (which can't run on ketones), need glucose, your body can supply the brain with all it needs through a process of gluconeogenesis. Your body reformulates the glycogen in your body to pull glycose out of it to use whenever the brain needs the glucose. (Remember, glycose used to be the name for glucose.)The interesting thing about this little-known fact is that your body makes this glucose, regardless of how much you already have in your body from the carbs you eat. This is one of the biggest benefits of ketosis, which we'll be talking about later.

This all points to the fact that your body will make the glucose it needs, provided you feed it the proper foods, to begin with, and carbs are not in that group. Carbs make your body make its own fat. It makes that fat out of the carbs you eat with the hormone insulin. (That's an enzyme you don't want to be inhibited.) A healthier way to live is to allow your body to make its own glucose instead of fat. This does wonders for the body. As long as you eat enough protein to compensate for the loss of muscle tissue from gluconeogenesis, you'll never lose vital muscle tissue.

This is why fasts help you lose so much weight. After your body uses up its own fat to fuel your body, it resets your body to produce growth hormones that not only help keep you thinner; they keep you healthier by repairing your systems for you (without the need for medication).

It does this by changing your hormones. The ways in which many hormones work are affected by eliminating carbs from the diet. Insulin is soon replaced by glucagon which regulates the gluconeogenesis that takes place in your body whenever it needs glucose. This hormone regulates how fat is **burned** in your body, whereas insulin controls how fat is stored in your body. As long as you're eating carbs you're creating insulin and it's instructing all the fat you're making, to be stored, instead of being used. When you remove the carbs from your body; your body changes, from increasing its production of insulin to increasing the production of glucagon which in turn ramps up the burning of your fat. This is why keto diets work so good. It's also why carb diets work so bad.

That means when you continue a diet of carbs, you're forcing your body to make its own fat out of those carbs and this is where your problem lies. The fat your body turns the glucose into is not a clean burning fat. It's a dirty fat at best. It leaves glycated residue wherever it's burned. That, in turn, gums up your cells...all of them, including your brain cells, your heart cells, your kidney cells, liver cells, every cell that blood flows through including the blood vessels they flow through. This is the true danger in carbohydrate consumption. This danger has been magnified by the glyphosate herbicide Roundup, with its enzyme inhibiting chemicals.

Some of the enzymes that get affected are enzymes that influence behavior. Some of these behavioral enzymes influence your appetite, as well as digestion, making this enzyme inhibitor responsible for more of your hunger and less of your nutrition. (It could actually detract from your nutrition.) It makes you hungrier, which in turn, can have an effect on your behavior. The behavior it tends to influence the most, is fear. I talk about that in Chapter 6.

Monsanto knows what enzymes their chemicals inhibit to have designed this weed killer. They have to know that these same enzymes are used in your body. They have to know how much this drives their pharmaceutical business. Could that be why Monsanto is so adamant about their product being safe? It's definitely not, and they know it. They engineered it. They know what enzymes it inhibits. They also know that those enzymes are used in the human body as well as plants. How can they possibly say that they can't add up this information to warn people of this danger? If you can answer this question, you can answer if this is really a ruse or not. I assure you, it is. It's too profitable to not be.

I'm sure, they have an idea, that cutting the use of enzyme inhibitors in crops will cut down on the need for the medication, the ingestion of those chemicals create, due to the changes those enzyme inhibitors impose on the body. This could be devastating for Monsanto. If news like that were to leak out to the world, they could lose millions, in profits in the pharmaceutical corporations they used to own?

You may not see any correlation yet, but I assure you, you will. What would happen to the profits of the food producers that depend on the grain industry to provide them with their flour, sugar, corn meal, and soy? Don't you think that would have a major influence on them if everyone knew that it was actually all of the grain products that Monsanto is responsible for, that is making them need the very medications that Monsanto's old pharmaceutical companies, make?

I'm sure the pharmaceutical companies are still customers of Monsanto chemical division now, buying the same enzyme inhibitors to use in heart medication as well as many cancer medications. This practice leads only to more and more drug need by their consumers and this is how you get hooked. If you eat grains in any form you're one of their consumers.

This is what happened to my mother and continues to happen to over 20,000 other mothers, every day across the world. This vicious cycle is courtesy of Monsanto's crop seed companies, Monsanto's herbicide companies through the production of Roundup, and what used to be Monsanto's corporate partner, Pharmacia (Pfizer and now Bayer, through their merger with Monsanto). In Europe and much of the rest of the world, it can be attributed to Syngenta, as well. They all own crop seed companies as well as pharmaceutical companies, as well as chemical companies to supply the pharmaceutical and crop seed companies. Are you alarmed, yet?

Cutting down on the use of these herbicides will also cut down on the need to use these same chemicals, they need, to produce those medicines and this is the doom they've condemned our society too. Their greed is more important to them than the health and safety of all America. Their glyphosate ensures this for Monsanto even after their patent expired. It also ensures that America is not free, but still under the control of this industry and Monsanto.

ACCORDING TO WIKIPEDIA; *glyphosate kills plants by interfering with the synthesis of the <u>aromatic</u> amino acids phenylalanine, tyrosine, and tryptophan. It does this by inhibiting the enzyme 5-enolpyruvylshikimate-3-phosphate synthase (epsps), which catalyzes the reaction of shikimate-3-phosphate (s3p) and phosphoenolpyruvate to form 5-enolpyruvyl-shikimate-3-phosphate (epsp). Glyphosate is absorbed through foliage and minimally through roots, meaning that it is only effective on actively growing plants and cannot prevent seeds from germinating. After application, glyphosate is readily transported around the plant to growing roots and leaves and this systemic activity is important for its effectiveness. Inhibiting the enzyme causes shikimate to accumulate in plant tissues and diverts energy and resources away* *from other processes. While growth stops within hours of application, it takes several days for the leaves to begin turning yellow.*

This process of killing plants, works just as well, on killing humans. It just does it slower because you don't get the massive dose the plant gets. Keep in mind, this stuff goes directly to the roots and foliage, making all vegetables it's sprayed on, tainted for consumption, as most edible vegetables are root vegetables and leaf vegetables. This would guarantee that this glyphosate gets into your diet if you eat vegetables. You might find some safety in GMO free veggies, but that's no guarantee.

This can make your body waste a lot more energy, converting those carbs into fat, so it can use them. If you feed your body fat in the first place, you don't need to convert anything as the fat is "ready to use". This last little factor is what's important to know because it doesn't require your body to make fat out of the sugar. This is what drains your pancreas from its supply of insulin. It also glycates your blood and it's this glycation, that leads to more modern disease than any other one thing. If you can control glycation, you control all inflammation. Controlling all inflammation means that you're controlling all modern diseases created by inflammation.

This fact combined with the fact that Roundup affects the enzymes **phenylalanine**, **tyrosine**, and **tryptophan**, means that they're also affecting your hunger patterns and your digestion. That creates a double dipper for the food industry and pharmaceutical industry. And they do this legally, thanks to a patent law from 1954 and a Supreme Court ruling that was written by an old Monsanto lawyer (Clearance Thomas) saying that modifying seeds for any purpose, is legal. I'm sure they didn't realize the consequences, at the time, their actions would have on humanity. The devastation it's created is monumental, in the least.

One of the enzymes affected in your body, Phenylalanine, is a precursor for **tyrosine**; the **monoamine neurotransmitters** for **dopamine**, norepinephrine (noradrenaline), and epinephrine (adrenaline); and the skin **pigment melanin**. Affecting phenylalanine is going to affect how your other hormones work that are influenced by these enzymes. Tryptophan is an enzyme that influences your hunger by influencing enzymes that affect hormones that are influenced by what you eat. This is why your hunger is greater now than it ever was in the past and this is why the obesity epidemic, diabetes epidemic, CVD epidemic, cancer epidemic and dementia epidemics have worsened alongside the increase of glyphosate sprayed on American crops. That means you must get your calories from healthier sources, like fats and protein. These are the foods your body prefers. It can live on carbs but carbs are only supposed to be used in times when we can't get the protein or fat.

The healthiest fats to partake of are MCT fats, Medium Chain Triglycerides. They'll balance your cholesterol which is much healthier than just lowering it. Balancing it will actually lower your LDL by increasing your HDL. It's the HDL that cleans out your cells of the spent LDL that was burned for fuel, from being fed into them. If your body can't clean out the burned LDL out of your cells, the LDL backs up in your blood increasing your overall cholesterol. What's worse? If you accumulated this LDL from eating carbs, it's dirty LDL, which is going to leave a residue inside your cells and this is what turns carbs into poison. That residue is what leads to all the modern diseases known to man. If you can cut down on that residue, you can control all disease. A simpler solution couldn't exist

Protein and fat have been the basis of our diet as far back as our species dates. We're not going to change that overnight by converting to a diet of carbs. That's insanity. Homo Sapiens went through well over 100,000 years eating protein and fat, supplementing it with carbs. Today, the basis of our diet is carbs and we supplement it with protein and fat. This practice urged on by a grain industry that's interested only in profits and not public health, has proven deadly for all Americans. Since the expansion of the use of Roundup, this practice has become the deadliest practice that mankind has been condemned to.

This weed killer has turned into a people killer, through its enzyme inhibiting functions and this is something Monsanto continues to deny. They've made lying to the public legal, with their placements in the USDA, FDA, EPA and probably the CDC all to ensure their success in carrying out their grandiose ruse that grains are healthy to eat and that you need to eat more of them. Hold on to that thought because we're going to look into why they're pushing this on the public like they are.

Thousands of years ago in our Paleolithic state, we were primarily carnivores. We've always had the ability to digest plant food but our bodies transformed to needing more protein to feed our growing brains, as we evolved over 6.8 millions years.

However, eating carbohydrates has its bad side, and it's called glycation. Protein can't create glycation. Fat can't create glycation. They both need the glucose to do that. That makes glucose a natural poison that we've been eating for over 10,000 years, only to be ramped up in the last 50 years or so to where the proliferation of its use is now sending hoards of people to their premature deaths. It's also making these same people very sick for extended periods of time before they die. It's making more and more people sick as they continue to eat, what now are really dirty carbs, due to the glyphosate herbicide sprayed on them as many as four times before they reach your table. Think about that for a minute.

The bread you make your sandwich with has been poisoned, right under your nose without your consent, or knowledge, which forces you to need the pharmaceuticals that this same company produces. Who knew that this addiction that's been forced upon you, claims your health, with every bite you take? You may, or may not, know what addiction this is by now and what you can do about it. What they're selling as safe, has escalated death rates from diabetes to brain cancer, from Alzheimer's to atherosclerosis, all evidenced by the rise in cancer rates in the farmers that use this weed killer on their crops. If you're not sure, read on.

It's evidenced by the rise in all major diseases since the start of spraying, 40 years ago. CVD rates climbed steadily for 15 – 20 years from the early 70's when they started using glyphosate, until they too, skyrocketed in the 90's when glyphosate usage multiplied. Now glyphosate is at an all-time high with every rate of modern disease at an all-time high as well. Yet Monsanto and its industry refuse to acknowledge the true damage they're doing to our society. It's their greed that's driving every pandemic known to modern man. From destroying our health to destroying the environment, Monsanto is leaving quite possibly, the largest footprint on our ecosystem, medical system, pharmaceutical system as well as our agricultural system. They have industrialized legal covert terrorism on an unsuspecting public, by saturating our diets with poisonous food, without telling us. What they should have shared with us, was that they were using us as guinea pigs, for their experiment on the impact glyphosate has on human physiology. In chapter 5 you'll see graphs for increase in autism.

Their experiment has been disastrous for the American people, as well as the world, as glyphosate is breaking records in sales every year, especially since the patent expired 16 years ago. But this isn't supposed to be about glyphosate. This is about the calories you eat and where you get them from. Do you get them from dirty sources like carbs or do you get them from efficient foods like protein and fats? An important thing to remember with your diet, a gram of sugar has 4 calories and a gram of fat has 9 calories? That points to the fact that fat is 225% more efficient as a food source. With fat being that much more efficient than sugar, it's no wonder that it's that much healthier.

Eating the proper fats feeds your body exactly what it's been running on ever since we've been running as a species. And run, we did in our Paleolithic years. We ran all day long, either hunting food, tracking down food, or just running down our food. The funny thing about this is, they were all running on empty stomachs, all day long, and not running out of energy. They could only do this by not eating many carbs. Their bodies had to run on ketones and fat, ramped up by adiponectin, testosterone, and other hormones in their bodies that set their brains to grow, faster and bigger.

It was this constant practice of exercising every day that made their bodies produce the hormones that allowed them to advance faster than the other species. It was our ability to sweat and cool our bodies that allowed our ancestors to run down their game to feed their families. It was this kind of diet that our bodies ate for 190,000 years.

10,000 years ago, we started cultivating this grain making it easier to collect and eat, making it a staple for the last 8,000+ years. Not until the last 60 years or so did we become so sedentary and start eating even more of what used to take us a half a day of gathering to eat. Most people now get their calories without the gathering or the hunting or the running so they never burn up those calories. They store them.

We're not as physically active as we were, even 50 years ago, and this where the problem starts. The same hormone, (insulin) instructs the fat it just made, to store itself as visceral fat around your midsection until you need it. Your problem is, you seldom need it, so it stays as fat. Even when you do need it, you seldom use all of what's available, so what you don't use stays as fat. This is the inherent problem with a carbohydrate diet, the need to make fat out of a sticky substance.

The bad thing about this process is that this fat you just made out of your carbs is going to demand more fat to join it. Fat in your body shuts down the action of leptin, the satiety hormone. When this hormone isn't working right to tell you when to put down your spoon, it's demanding that your body consume more carbs to satisfy it. This leptin resistance leads directly to your need, to eat more and more, just to produce enough leptin to satisfy your addiction. And this is precisely why you should get your calories from protein and a much more efficient fat, rather than carbs. (This is why modern disease has become more pervasive in the last 7,000 years. We exchanged the easy pickings and safety of not having, to risk being prey, to hunt, which is what killed most prehistoric men, for the unknown dangers of glycation and glucose addiction. This may have saved our species for 7,000 years, but it's killing us in hordes, currently.)

This Leptin resistance is Metabolic Syndrome, a precursor to diabetes. This is one reason the keto diet is taking off so much. It's not only a fat burning diet, it's a brain growing, muscle growing diet that truly gives you the best body and brain you can have. Nobody, on a ketogenic diet has ever gotten diabetes.

You should be asking yourself, what kind of fat is good to eat? We've always been told that fat is bad. Until I learned that it isn't, I thought the same thing. It's actually healthy, truthfully, it's very healthy. The industry that told you it was bad, had an interest in selling you that idea, so you would eat more carbs. They even recommended for you to eat them over the fat. That's because the grain industry is behind the recommendations for what you eat and their interest is in supplying more grains for you to consume.

Later, they found out that a diet of fat won't lead you to any drug use. That's reserved for the carb diet and that may have been why this industry dissuaded everyone from consuming a diet of fat. This is something Monsanto has lied to you about, for over 40 years. Just like the sugar industry the grain industry has been lying to the public for greater than 60 years about the safety in eating their food. Now, they've amplified its danger by dousing it with more and more glyphosate right up until two weeks before harvest. How safe do you think that makes the food you eat?

Remember the thought I asked you to hold on to earlier, why Monsanto has been pushing the idea that grains are healthy to eat? The answer to that question is multifaceted because this is a crop that can be marketed to farmers as making them more money by producing more crop. Yet they need to spread more Roundup, to do this, according to Monsanto. (This is something many farmers don't agree with and are actively trying to resist. Monsanto's push to own every farmer on North American soil has taken many of these farmers to court where Monsanto has tied them up for years at a time, often, to get them to use their own GMO seed.) This includes Canada where a majority of canola is grown, which happens to be another Monsanto glyphosated crop (rapeseed). This is another one that they like to spray with Roundup right before harvesting to save the lower oil pods that drop off the crop and shatter losing much of the valuable canola oil. For the farmer, it's Roundup to the rescue. For the consumer, it's Roundup to the dinner table where it can continue its enzyme inhibiting actions in the bodies of your family. That consequence of its use leads to purchase of these same chemicals in medications to counteract the damage created by them, in the first place.

Right after Monsanto patented their first seed in 1980, they purchased GD Searle chemicals, maker of NutraSweet, in 1985. This was about 14 years after they patented Roundup. Their Roundup has done a bang-up job of bringing the senescence of glyphosate to humans. Roundup is advertised as working through senescence, on how it kills weeds. That senescence is rubbing off on our population. It was 7 years after they patented seeds that they patented Celebrex, setting themselves up to be a provider of foods that require an early departure to drugs and a never-ending cycle of drug use that never lets up until a premature death.

This current cycle of disease, disorder, and death can be traced back to 1954 and the plant act. That's when they made it legal to patent seeds, later leading to genetic modifying of crop seed, later leading to genetically modifying crop seed to survive multiple uses of an enzyme inhibiting herbicide that induces senescence in humans. This is how the genetic modifying of humans by modifying their food, evolved. This food that gets modified just happens to be an addictive food that's been made more addictive by its modifying. If this isn't criminal in nature, I don't know what is.

To prevent your premature death, look to make fat and protein the core of your diet. You don't have to eat nearly as much, or as often, as it's that dreaded hunger cycle that never appears in the keto diet. That's because the arguably worst manifestation of a carbohydrate diet, is the hunger cycle that's tied to it. I don't know anyone who would want that (except for an addict). Especially when that hunger gets magnified by what's been sprayed on it multiple times. It helps to understand this if you're already on a keto diet and have broken the addiction.

It's clear to me that the more glyphosate that Monsanto sells, the more disease the public is going to fight. From autism to Alzheimer's, all modern diseases have increased right alongside the increase of glyphosate usage. The only blessing here, is that we don't have to eat it. We can say no to glyphosate, by not eating any grains, including sugar.

Carbohydrates The unsustainable food source.

By using carbs/glucose for daily caloric intake, you set yourself up for needing more and more carbs to keep up the same amount of energy. The cycle is completely unsustainable because the desire for carbs far precedes the need for them.

Long before your last meal is even digested, your body releases ghrelin, the hormone that signals to your stomach that you're hungry, telling your brain that it's time to eat again. This is also your growth hormone. The opposite to this hormone is leptin, your satiety hormone, it's the one that tells you when to put your fork down.

It's this hormone that's dangerous, as this is a hormone of fat storage. When extra visceral fat lies around the mid-section, this hormone, leptin takes up residence in it. The problem is, as soon as your stomach starts to shrink, this signals the brain to trigger the ghrelin, signaling that you're hungry again, demanding more of the "carb made" fat, where the leptin resides. It's the worst *"catch 22"* you can get caught up in.

The inherent problem with carbs is that they need insulin to digest them. Insulin is the ultimate fat building hormone. All fat, created by insulin is instructed by that hormone, to go to storage. If your body can't produce enough insulin for your diet, it's past time to change your diet to one where you won't need the insulin, a diet without carbs.

If you're not eating carbs, you're not using insulin and insulin is the fat hormone. As long as you're using it, you're adding fat to your body that doesn't get used until your stomach is empty and glucagon is generated to burn up that fat. That's the basis of why the Glucose Ruse works so well. Fat is a self-feeding disease that must keep building itself up, more and more until you have obesity and diabetes, then heart disease, or cancer. You will suffer arthritis, atherosclerosis, to some extent, high blood pressure (that's virtually guaranteed). Diabetes always comes. I know. It runs in my family. My grandfather had it, my sisters had it, my father struggles with it.
That's because my mother, in trying to do her best for her family, fed us these grains in the amounts that were recommended by our USDA and FDA and even the ADA. Yeah, the ADA, American Dietary Association recommends them. Why? When they cause so much damage, why would they recommend them? Who would profit off of that? The pharmaceutical industry? The chemical industry? The food industry? The beverage industry?

Who's money are they taking though? Who buys their groceries? Who eats their grains? Who buys their medicines? If you eat this food, you buy into this ruse. It's easy to do, really easy. It is addictive, after-all. Their job is half done for them. All they have to do is find companies to make products and promote them, like soda, beer, and wine, bread, pasta, breakfast cereals and pastries. This is where it where it bites you the worst, because we're all born into it, so it's already started by the time we're born.

All of our baby food reinforces our addiction by pumping more glucose into our bodies as it's in almost all baby food and formula. It's in almost all OTC baby medicines. Have you ever tried to find any baby medicine without high fructose corn syrup as its primary ingredient? It's impossible.

Why wouldn't an industry dependent on your addiction for their survival, (as their industry was built on your addiction), want to keep you addicted? Their money is tied up in your addiction. The more you eat of their products, the more of their medicines, you'll be buying. Welcome to the Glucose Ruse.

We know, now, that carbs are what creates the fat, that we don't use until our stomach is empty. Why, do we still eat them to excess, then? In one word, addiction. It's this addiction that leads to its worst manifestation, and that's glycation, the foundation of all disease. The ultimate effect of any addiction is disease and death and it's no different with carb addiction. It just takes longer than all other addictions. That's why these industries use this addiction to take the money of those who buy into it.

We haven't even looked at the amount of land taken up by industrial farming that's contributing to global warming as well as being the foundation of this Glucose Ruse, putting Monsanto, now Bayer, at the core of this ruse. Ever since Bayer merged with Monsanto to take over the chemical company, our food production is under the control of an eastern European country, Germany, since Bayer is a German company.

If I still ate any grains, I'd be concerned. I'd be concerned, big-time, about this development in the production of my food. Wasn't it Stalin who said, control the food, you control the people. Yeah! I'd be concerned...but, I don't eat them, so I'm not as concerned about what's in them as you should be, because I don't eat them, although, I am concerned about what they're feeding everybody else and unfortunately, 87% of us are still addicted. That concerns me. As long as this addiction continues, diseases will continue. That, to me, is not acceptable.

How much of the health industry is dependent on our obesity? How much do we spend to lose weight or stay healthy, or worse yet, how much do we spend trying to regain our health, after we lose it? That's why the pharmaceutical industry is reaping such profits from those of us who're still buying into it? How much money do we spend fighting cancer? How much is spent on therapies? Therapy for any of a myriad of physical disabilities caused by degeneration of bone tissue and arthritis, both rheumatoid and osteoarthritis would not exist if it weren't for our carbohydrate diet.

What companies make up the biggest portion of those who sell the most dangerous foods? What are the most dangerous foods? We already know that the problem lies in grain ingestion, which includes sugar, as sugar is a grain, sugar cane. There are several industries built around the celebration of this addiction. From several snack companies, as well as several beverage companies including, several beer and wine companies, as well as all bakeries and bakery corporations. The list of corporations in these industries is, truly endless.

THE PAIN THAT MAKES YOU LAME
AND DRAINS YOUR BRAIN
COMES MAINLY
FROM THE GRAINS
FROM THE PLAINS
IT'S THE GLUCOSE RUSE
THAT BRINGS YOUR BLUES
WHICH WILL BE WHAT YOU ETERNALLY RUE
FROM THE TIME YOU ATE THAT GLUE
THAT MAKES YOU PAY THOSE UGLY DUES

III
Your Celebration of Your Addiction to Sugar, and the Price You Pay For It.
Carbohydrates and their Lure

It's not hard to see how much you enjoy, celebrating your addiction to carbs. It's displayed in everything that's said and done, in all aspects of the food industry. It's boldly advertised everywhere you go. What you don't know is that addiction is a complete surrender to sugar and carbs. Shortly following this celebration of addiction that you love to express, comes a parade of drugs that you'll be taking, to treat all of the symptoms that come from succumbing to your addiction. This simple equation, requires that we curb the influence, of the grain and pharmaceutical industry, on our health.

Failure to control this influence will, not only lead to more disease and illness, but more, to greater health costs overall. How are we ever going to put an end to diabetes? Or an end to Alzheimer's disease? Or cancer? Or heart disease? Or arthritis? Or hypertension? Hyperlipidemia or High Cholesterol? How are we ever going to learn to live healthily and kick this habit, before it destroys our society?

I would like to show just how our celebration of our addiction to sugar is not only destroying our individual lives, it has the possibility of destroying our entire civilization, if we don't curb its influence, and the most devastating influence this has on our society, is displayed by the amount of fear, it's increased, since its usage, increased. Want to know, where the terrorism really comes from? That's in chapter 6, *The Real Reason for Terrorism and War*. Don't forget what Stalin said about controlling the people by controlling their food. You might want to keep that in mind as you read the rest of this story.

I intend to show you how this industry hooks you in the first place, how they keep you hooked, so in the future, you're forced to buy into their drug habit. This drug habit involves anti-inflammatories like NSAIDS (aspirin, Motrin, Advil, Aleve), Tylenol, antacids, anti-gas and bloating, (Pepto Bismol, Gaviscon, Alka Seltzer) and we're just starting with the OCDs. For prescription medicine, we're looking at all opioids (Oxycontin, Oxycodone, Vicodin, Percocet), which again are addictive. More prescription NSAIDS like Celebrex, Relafen, Relifex, and Gambaran. We know that by the existing opioid abuse epidemic how dangerous these drugs are. Do you think this happened by chance?

Other prescription medicines that you're doomed to need if you continue your carbohydrate consumption (especially for those who allow ECC to control them), includes but are not limited to; statins, **vasoactive** agents, **fibrates**, and **CETP Inhibitors**, just for starters. Statins are, by far, the far worst of these medications.

After spending 15 years giving care to and for seniors, I have seen the ravages statin drugs have taken on their bodies. They slowly rob their users from their mental faculties, then their muscles, then their lives. This proves the importance of cholesterol and how much it influences. What it takes away from its users is in no way replaced by the treatment it offers. They are nothing more than invitations to a need to take more and more drugs. Is there a reason that the drug industry has found ways to make you buy more of their wares?

I've only talked about heart medications so far, I haven't even touched on cancer medication or cholesterol medication (many of which are related to heart medications like statins), nor have I covered other prescription medication for Alzheimer's disease, high blood pressure, and Parkinson's. The list goes on and on. What a quagmire this has turned out to be. You'll be interested in how to get yourself out it. I'll cover that, starting in Chapter 10.

Cholesterol, your body's fuel

The pharmaceutical industry wants you to think that high cholesterol has something to do with heart disease, which couldn't be further from the truth and that high cholesterol is dangerous. This is absolutely false. Cholesterol isn't the problem. Cholesterol is healthy. Your body has to use it to stay alive. Taking cholesterol away from your body takes away your body's fuel source and only leads to more medication. This is devastating for you. I can see where this would benefit the drug industry, though. Is that where your savings are earmarked for? Or are you relying on insurance to cover your expenses? Got co-pays? I've learned that they add up quickly, especially when it comes to meds, meds and more meds. How many do you currently take? Is that an expense you could do without?

High cholesterol isn't a heart problem. It's a diet problem. Your diet is responsible for your high cholesterol. Your major food source is your primary source of cholesterol and that is where the problem begins. Your high carbohydrate diet produces cholesterol in your body that is not clean cholesterol, meaning that it is dirty fuel, as cholesterol is your body's fuel. This is cholesterol you don't need. You need clean cholesterol that's been produced by fat. That is what powers our bodies. With clean cholesterol, your body functions perfectly, because chances are, if your cholesterol is clean, it's come from sources that are clean, and that's directly from fat and high cholesterol foods, like eggs. Low cholesterol is a recipe for poor health, as too much of your health comes from cholesterol.

Cholesterol is your body's fuel source. It's cholesterol that enters the cell to be burned as fuel, so what's important is the kind of cholesterol that your body uses. Is it clean, or dirty cholesterol? Cholesterol from carbohydrates, is a dirty sticky fuel, due to the nature of what this cholesterol comes from. It comes from a sticky, icky, gooey, gluey substance, sugar and its residue after it's burned is just as sticky. This is what leads to plaque, the basis of almost all cancers, heart diseases and all dementias.

I prove in the next chapter how the discontinuance of these foods leads only to better health and how continued consumption of these foods, only leads to a path of illness and disease. What I don't know, did this industry know what these foods do from the studies that have come out over the last 70+ years? Or did they remain electively ignorant of the reports? Or did they influence the cover-up of these reports? With as many reports that have come out, I have to wonder. There are just so many of them (11,222) that it's easy to mess with a lot of them. Later I'll show you how this industry has had its problems in the courts. Some of it is not pretty. I'll list just a few of the studies that have shown this damage going back over 70 years. The earliest study I found in 11,222 studies done over the years, that mentioned, glycation is dangerous, was completed in 1960. In this study, they linked diabetes with atherosclerosis. I looked through page after page of studies that started in the 60's, 70's & the 80's. They seem to grow in number as time goes on. Studies have exploded since the turn of this century, as more and more people are starting to recognize the true dangers this food imposes on its consumers. Yet the majority of the addicted choose to remain ignorant of its dangers, as they're impotent in ignoring its lures. They are all controlled by their hormones which are controlling their emotions. This is a common trait of carbolism. The addicted have little to no choice in the matter. The need to feed the addiction is no less than that of any other addiction, which forces the addicted to continue to feed the addiction. It's the way addiction works, it's the way carbolism works.

Celebration of addiction

We're inundated with the commercialism of addiction on a daily basis. You see advertising for these foods and drinks everywhere. How many snack food companies are there? How many cereal companies are there? How many soft drink companies are there? How many beer and spirits companies, are there? How many commercials do you see each day from these industries? All of those commercials are luring you into their web of addiction. The grain industry has found ways to infect our society, like cockroaches in a garbage pit.

We all know who profits from this today, but have you ever connected that with who is going to profit from it 10, 20, 30 years from now, the pharmaceutical industry? It seems that the grain industry's intent is to do nothing more than to fuel the drug industry. Whether it is their intent or not, it is and has been the result. How long it continues to be, depends on how long we continue to allow our addictions to exist.

Drug companies, right now, are foaming at the mouth for all the business the food industry has sent them. Nobody is interested in breaking this addiction. What more could they ask for, a captive audience, all set up to need what they have, to feed your addiction at a cost that they set. You get to pay it or deal with your pain. Many times you have to pay it, just to stay alive. Do you wonder why medical costs keep going up or why insurance costs so much? If everyone would stop buying into this ruse and find their cure, what would happen to the pharmaceutical industry? A huge drop in demand for their drugs would lower the price for the drugs as well as the treatments. It's not hard to see the benefit that would have.

The underlying cause of addiction

First off, let's define addiction. Dictionary.com defines addiction; *noun: the state of being enslaved to a habit or practice or to something that is psychologically or physically habit-forming, as narcotics, to such an extent that its cessation causes severe trauma."*

I differentiate mental habit from a physical addiction. Where an addiction presents a physical need, a habit only creates a psychological need. The difference is in what the body demands and what the mind demands, and where discomfort, plays into the equation. Is it a physical discomfort or just a mental discomfort?

Wikipedia defines *addiction;* "*Addiction is a medical condition characterized by compulsive engagement in rewarding stimuli, despite adverse consequences.*"

I personally define addiction as a compulsion to consume a substance that the body craves but doesn't need, as it actually harms the body. All of these definitions ring true for heroin and opioids, sugar and alcohol, cigarettes and tobacco, The three most abused substances in the civilized algorithm, although not in that order. The worst of these addictions is that of sugar and alcohol, with sugar being by far, the meanest and vilest scourge ever committed upon the human race.

It basically starts while we're in our mother's womb, as fetuses. Our nutrition comes from her blood, which always has a certain amount of glucose in it due the bread, pasta, and cereal she's eaten while pregnant. All that glucose she's eating is what you ate and got addicted to.

Then it continues with sugar and carbs in the baby food. It's obvious why they put it in baby food. That's because it's so palatable and goes down so easy. What baby doesn't love the taste of sugar? This taste for sugar is your first indication of the addiction, requiring it be fed every other hour or so. Whether or not this was the intended consequences of the marketing of this food, this consequence has become America's newest death sentence. By showing how this addiction affects the body in the next chapter, *THE DANGERS OF GLYCATION,* the evidence proves how dangerous this food is to human physiology. Yet we continue to celebrate our addiction to it.

The major reason this addiction continues is due to the manner in which it is, and has been promoted. The desire to create more and more ways and forms to entice everyone to eat and drink more of this deadly food is nothing short of astounding. It continues to amaze me how inventive we are at finding ways to kill ourselves with our own taste buds. Studies have been done, books have been written, the public has been warned, but it continues to happen. Every time I turn around I see another new way to kill ourselves in another appealing commercial. All this advertising encouraging us to consume more and more of their blood glucose raising, diabetes causing, HBP causing, dementia-causing foods is the driving force of this addiction and consequent expense.

A carbohydrate diet requires that you feed it almost on an hourly basis. A ketogenic diet, on the other hand, allows you to go all day without eating much of anything. Here's the secret, carboholics don't like to go without food. They do almost anything they can to not go hungry. Those on a ketogenic diet, don't mind going without food. To us, it's not going hungry. It's simply going without eating. The hunger doesn't exist as much, as the cycle of addiction has been broken. We feel the hunger pangs and many times, welcome them because we know that is where we build our better health. We do this by building Ghrelin throughout our systems because we know that Ghrelin works to build our immunity as well as making us a little smarter by increasing our brain power, through the addition of BDNF in our brains. As explained in *It's Time for a Cure,* BDNF is that stuff that's the foundation of new brain cells. Don't forget the Nrf2, that ramps up the production of your anti-oxidants. Those are both benefits of Ghrelin in your system.

Your celebration of your addiction to this sugar is the industry's celebration of profits, both in the food, they sell us and the drugs we buy to relieve the pain. For them, it's a win-win situation. For the public who buys into this, it's a no-win situation. This is the prescription for future medications if you're in your teens and twenties. In your thirties, you'll start buying their headache and stomach ache medication. In your forties, it'll become insulin or anti-diabetes medication, then in your 50's and 60's and beyond, pick your poison, heart disease, cancer, Alzheimer's disease. Anyone or all of these are going to hit you when you least expect it.

Targeted Advertising

Almost everything I see advertised on channels marketing to younger viewers, is encouraging everyone to buy more cereal, soda, energy drinks (most of which are laden with sugar), power bars, snack chips and cereals. Then, when you're a few years older, the ads are aimed at selling you pizza and beer. Then into your 40's, 50's and 60's the ads are all aimed at selling you treatments and drugs for all the diseases and illnesses that your lifetime of consumption has brought you, drugs for diabetes, heart disease, cancer, arthritis, dementia, HPB, high cholesterol, etc, etc. How long do I need to go on? Did I mention headaches or stomach aches?

When I watch programming on TV appealing to older viewers, like news broadcasts, I'm inundated with the commercials they show for drugs to treat heart disease (for which, there is no cure, only treatment), to treat cancer (again no cure), diabetes, high cholesterol, high blood pressure, arthritis, diabetes, and obesity. Drug companies are doing their best to sell their drugs to us, to treat (not cure) us, for the illness and pain that they cause. And we buy it. We buy into it big time. We've bought into it our entire lives. The biggest problem here is most people are still buying into it. And they're buying into it in massive quantities, evidenced by the pandemics of obesity, diabetes, Alzheimer's disease, heart disease, cancer, arthritis, HBP, etc, etc. What's being spent now, not just on snacks and beverages, but on staples like flour and sugar, pasta and cereal will be tripled, quadrupled, quintupled and even more, in payments to the pharmaceutical companies in the future, after you're done paying the price, for the damage, all your years of consumption will cause. The only way to getting as close to a cure, as you can, is to give them up as completely as possible, otherwise, continuing will only incur the need for drugs.

The drugs they'll be pushing on you, for heart disease or cancer, or even just for your headaches and stomach aches will be an array of **SIDE EFFECT** causing chemicals that will ultimately make it necessary for you to purchase more of their drugs to counteract the side effects of the drugs you've been taking for your treatment. You see proof of this everywhere. I experienced it myself when I was on 12 different medications just to treat an underlying chronic pain problem. I had to take diuretics for my high blood pressure, anti-depressants because "they worked on the same receptors in the brain that the pain used", NSAIDS for the headaches I always used to get, opioids for the chronic pain I live with from the car accident. The diuretics were for my high blood pressure caused by my pain, or so I thought. After I quit the bread, the pain subsided. Maybe not completely, but enough to encourage me to quit all grains. When it subsided, even more, I decided to quit all carbs. My biggest benefit was the loss of my high blood pressure along with 30 lbs of weight.

When they advertise new drugs, the precautions and side effects of the drugs they want to sell you, take up more of the commercials, they show, than the explanations of their benefits. I have to wonder where the regulation is. Is it for the consumer (which it's supposed to be) or is this regulation for the benefit of the industry? How can drugs with that many precautions and side effects still be approved for sale? It appears to me that this industry has the FDA under their spell.

Which does it appear to be, to you? This industry is still allowed to market foods of disease and death while marketing treatments for those diseases and illnesses. Who knew that these industries are related? Before I started this, I didn't. I had to uncover this information, so I'll show you how all this is connected and it's connected to take your money. Their manner of taking your money is clearly hazardous to your health. This is something you need to know because nothing is more important than your health.

The industry that feeds you, forces you to buy their drugs.

The food industry which also includes the grain industry, which includes the crop seed industry that provides the farmers with the seed they need to grow the grains that they sell us to put on our tables for us to eat, is related to the pharmaceutical industry that makes all the drugs for all the diseases that these foods create. My question is how could we allow an industry responsible for our food, be also responsible for the diseases their food creates?

What we've allowed these related industries to do, in a nutshell, is drain our wallets at the grocery store by influencing us to buy their hunger inducing, cereals, sodas, fruit drinks, snack foods, power bars, pastas, breads, granolas, cereals and crackers, while draining our wallets again, at the pharmacy to buy their drugs that treat the symptoms of the diseases their food is responsible for. I know. I've experienced it. I pray that you heed my words and don't experience it yourselves.

For the food, we're sold through their marketing....(and their advertising is pure magic to see and it's so easy to buy into), those of us that aren't aware, are buying into a lifetime of distress. Their product tastes better than anything in the world. How much more could you ask for than a worldwide customer base that's addicted to your wares? Because it's addictive (like tobacco), you only have to make it more appealing than that of its competitors, of which it has plenty because the addiction is so strong. That makes it deadlier than heroin, simply because it's as prevalent as water. In some places, more prevalent.

We also get to pay their associates for the drugs we need to combat the diseases that their food has given us. And pay them we do. We'll pay them anything to get out of the pain that we've been inflicted with, from eating the food they so happily sold to us. We just don't connect that pain we feel with the food we've grown up with. But it is connected. It's connected in a big way. They first connected themselves toward the end of the 20th century with mergers and acquisitions bringing chemical, pharmaceutical, and crop seed companies under one name, Monsanto.

The Perfect Ruse

This disturbs me and it disturbs me immensely. The company that produces the crop seed for the food I'm supposedly going to eat is the same pharmaceutical company that makes drugs for the illnesses and diseases this food is responsible for? Is it legal? It isn't illegal. It happens and you buy into it.

This industry is so intent on keeping us addicted that sugar or corn syrup is quite often the #1 or #2 ingredient in baby food, meaning that if you're not, one of the few that are raised on their mother's milk and had to grow up on baby food, you're condemned to an addiction that our grain and pharmaceutical industry has imposed upon you.

It's not surprising that we've ignored this addiction for as long as we've had it. We've ignored it because we grew up with it. Everyone has it, so as far as everyone is concerned, there is no addiction. After all, how can you be addicted to something that you need to survive? How can you live without something that you need to survive? That's where the question lies, in whether or not, it's something you need to survive. Do you really need this food or can you live without it?

If you take anything from this book, let this be at the heart of what you take. You can live without carbs and you should live without carbs. To do this, you make your body not need carbs. Sounds simple, doesn't it? It is simple, it just isn't easy. This is one case where simple is not easy.

We've made it so easy for this industry to increase our addiction that we look forward to finding new ways to inflict more harm on our bodies. And this industry is more than happy to oblige us with their new creations to further our addiction. It's a win-win situation for them. They couldn't ask for anything more. We're paying one side for what we eat, while we pay the other side for drugs. Monsanto has made a fortune off of us, doing this. And we gladly give it to them, just to feed the addiction, we're born with that they propitiate.

Monsanto's involvement

According to Wikipedia; "*Monsanto scientists were among the first to genetically modify a plant cell, publishing their results in 1983; five years later, the company conducted the first field tests of genetically engineered crops. Increasing involvement in agricultural biotechnology R&D in general dates from the installment of Richard Mahoney as Monsanto's CEO in 1983. This involvement increased under the leadership of Robert Shapiro, appointed CEO in 1995, leading ultimately to divestment of product lines unrelated to agriculture*".

This divestment of product lines allowed their introduction into pharmaceuticals. Did they know at this time, what their food was doing to their consumers? Had they seen any of the reports that started coming out in 1960 and continued until today? Are they aware of any of them now? It appears not, or they're choosing to be electively ignorant. I suspect they have to be aware.

From Wikipedia; "*In 1985, Monsanto acquired G. D. Searle & Company, a life sciences company focusing on pharmaceuticals, agriculture, and animal health. In 1993, Monsanto's Searle division filed a patent application for Celebrex, which in 1998, became the first selectiveCOX-2 inhibitor to be approved by the U.S. Food and Drug Administration (FDA). Celebrex became a blockbuster drug and was often mentioned as a key reason for Pfizer's acquisition of Monsanto's pharmaceutical business in 2002.*"

Celebrex and arthritis, did they know the connection? What causes arthritis? Was this industry aware of the studies that started coming out in the 50's and 60's about the dangers of their food products and the glycation they caused? Any educated person, would think so. I'm not educated, but I think so.

- *"In 1996, Monsanto purchased Agracetus, the biotechnology company that had generated the first transgenic varieties of cotton, soybeans, peanuts, and other crops, and from which Monsanto had already been licensing technology since 1991. Monsanto first entered the maize seed business when it purchased 40% of DEKALB in 1996; it purchased the remainder of the corporation in 1998. In 1998 Monsanto purchased Cargill's international seed business, which gave it access to sales and distribution facilities in 51 countries. In 2005, it finalized the purchase of Seminis Inc, a leading global vegetable and fruit seed company, for $1.4 billion.*

This made it the world's largest conventional seed company at the time. Again, I have to wonder if they had seen the studies of what their products were doing to their consumers? That, makes me wonder, was this an intentional move to sell more pharmaceuticals? What corporation wouldn't avail themselves. of a chance like this? Most corporate bylaws, say, they must.

"In 2007, Monsanto and BASF announced a long-term agreement to cooperate in the research, development, and marketing of new plant biotechnology products." "Through a series of transactions, the Monsanto that existed from 1901 to 2000 and the current Monsanto are legally two distinct corporations. Although they share the same name and corporate headquarters, many of the same executives and other employees, and responsibility for liabilities arising out of activities in the industrial chemical business, the agricultural chemicals business is the only segment carried forward from the pre-1997 Monsanto Company to the current Monsanto Company. This was accomplished beginning in the 1980s:
- *1985: Monsanto purchased D. Searle & Company for $2.7 billion in cash. In this merger, Searle's aspartame business became a separate Monsanto subsidiary,*

- the NutraSweet Company. CEO of NutraSweet, Robert B. Shapiro, served as CEO of Monsanto from 1995 to 2001.
- *1996:* Monsanto acquired Agracetus, a majority interest in Calgene, creators of the Flavr Savr tomato, and 40% of DeKalb Genetics Corporation. It purchased the remainder of DeKalb in 1998.
- *1997:* Monsanto spun off its industrial chemical and fiber divisions into Solutia. In January, Monsanto announced the purchase of Holden's Foundations Seeds, a privately held seed business. By acquiring Holden's, Monsanto became the biggest American producer of foundation corn, the parent seed from which hybrids are made. The combined purchase price was $925 million. Also, in April, Monsanto purchased the remaining shares of Calgene.
- *1999:* Monsanto sold off NutraSweet Co. In December, Monsanto merged with Pharmacia & Upjohn, and the agricultural division became a wholly owned subsidiary of the "new" Pharmacia; the medical research divisions of Monsanto, which included products such as Celebrex, were rolled into Pharmacia. Sounds like the perfect match for a corruptible, collaboration of collusion, willing to take Stalin's notion, to test.
- *2000 (October):* Pharmacia spun off its Monsanto subsidiary into a new company, the "new Monsanto". Monsanto agreed to indemnify Pharmacia against any liabilities that might be incurred from judgments against Solutia. As a result, the new Monsanto continues to be a party to numerous lawsuits that relate to operations of the old Monsanto. Now, they're mired in lawsuits by farmers and crop dusters, filing countless lawsuits for cancer, due to the handling of their glyphosate. *Pharmacia was bought by Pfizer in a deal announced in 2002 and completed in 2003.)*
- *2005:* Monsanto acquired Emergent Genetics and its Stoneville and NexGen cotton brands. Emergent was the third largest U.S. cotton seed company, with about 12 percent of the U.S. market. Monsanto's goal was to obtain "a strategic cotton germ plasm and traits platform." The vegetable seed producer Seminis was purchased for $1.4 billion.
- *2007:* In June, Monsanto purchased Delta & Pine Land Company, a major cotton seed breeder, for $1.5 billion. As a condition for approval from the Department of Justice,

Monsanto was obligated to divest its Stoneville cotton business, which it sold to Bayer, and to divest its NexGen cotton business, which it sold to Americot. Monsanto also exited the pig breeding business by selling Monsanto Choice Genetics to Newsham Genetics LC in November, divesting itself of "any and all swine-related patents, patent applications, and all other intellectual property"

- *2008: Monsanto purchased the Dutch seed company De Ruiter Seeds for €546 million, and sold its POSILAC bovine somatotropin brand and related business to Elanco Animal Health, a division of Eli Lilly in August for $300 million plus "additional contingent consideration".*
- *2012: Monsanto purchased for $210 million Precision Planting Inc., a company that produced computer hardware and software designed to enable farmers to increase yield and productivity through more accurate planting.*
- *2013: Monsanto purchased San Francisco-based Climate Corp for $930 million Climate Corp. makes more accurate local weather forecasts for farmers based on data modeling and historical data; if the forecasts were wrong, the farmer was recompensed.*
- *2015 Monsanto tried to buy Syngenta for US$46.5 billion but failed.*
- *2016 Bayer offered to buy Monsanto for US$62 billion."*
- *2017 Bayer buys Monsanto*

Monsanto's involvement in the pharmaceutical industry and the agro sciences has grown to monopolistic proportions. It not only controls what goes into your food, but what you take for the diseases that food gives you.

It's not just crop seed that they manufacture; they also, are responsible for the chemicals sprayed on the crops grown from their seed. Since it's been genetically modified to withstand the effects of their herbicide, roundup, I've always wondered how much of those chemicals get into our food through this process. We know that Roundup is a glyphosate herbicide, meaning that it's an enzyme inhibitor, that's not good for human health. For me, it's just not healthy enough, especially for the problems I already live with. More chemicals in my body are not what I need to keep it healthy. You may want to take that chance, but pesticides and herbicides in our diet have been linked to bladder cancer. Why would I want to chance that, just for the taste of something sweet or salty? Any craving for salt is actually a craving for the carbs that come with the salt. The salt isn't addictive, the carbs are. Evidenced below is just a little of Monsanto's bio-chemical industry.

How glyphosate-based herbicides & GM seed combine to make consumption of grains dangerous.

Because they're so good at manufacturing the chemicals for the herbicides and pesticides, they manufacture GMO seed that is resistant to these chemicals. Though the plant may be resistant to the chemicals, does that mean that your body is? I don't think so.

Again according to Wikipedia; *"Monsanto chemist John E. Franz repurposed the chemical glyphosate as a systemic herbicide in 1970. Monsanto's last commercially relevant United States patent on glyphosate expired in 2000, and since then glyphosate has been marketed in the United States and worldwide by many agro-chemical companies, in different solution strengths, and with various adjuvants, under dozens of trade names. As of 2009, sales of glyphosate represented about 10% of Monsanto's revenue due to competition from other producers of other glyphosate-based herbicides; their Roundup products (which include GM seeds) represented about half of Monsanto's gross margin"*

Glyphosate is an enzyme inhibitor, used not only in herbicides but also in many drugs, as they're used as enzyme inhibitors in multiple forms of medications. They allow the drug to be more specific to the treatment, to incur fewer side effects, for the patient. This may be healthier for the patient who takes this drug, but, what if you never needed to take it?

What Wikipedia says about glyphosate; *"Glyphosate is absorbed through foliage, and minimally through roots, and transported to growing points. It inhibits a plant enzyme involved in the synthesis of three aromatic amino acids: tyrosine, tryptophan, and phenylalanine. Therefore, it is effective only on actively growing plants and is not effective as a pre-emergence herbicide. An increasing number of crops have been genetically engineered to be tolerant of glyphosate (e.g. Roundup Ready soybean, the first Roundup Ready crop, also created by Monsanto) which allows farmers to use glyphosate as a post-emergence herbicide against weeds. The development of glyphosate resistance in weed species is emerging as a costly problem. While glyphosate and formulations such as Roundup have been approved by regulatory bodies worldwide, concerns about their effects on humans and the environment persist."*

"Many regulatory and scholarly reviews have evaluated the relative toxicity of glyphosate as an herbicide. The German Federal Institute for Risk Assessment toxicology review in 2013 found that "the available data is contradictory and far from being convincing" with regard to correlations between exposure to glyphosate formulations and risk of various cancers, including non-Hodgkin lymphoma (NHL).

A 2014 review article reported a *"significant association between B-cell lymphoma and glyphosate occupational exposure. In March 2015 the World Health Organization's International Agency for Research on Cancer classified glyphosate as "probably carcinogenic in humans" (category 2A) based on epidemiological studies, animal studies, and in vitro studies. However in 2016 a joint meeting of the United Nations (FAO) Panel of Experts on Pesticide Residues in Food and the Environment and the World Health Organization (WHO) Core Assessment Group on Pesticide Residues (JMPR) concluded that based on the available evidence "glyphosate is unlikely to pose a carcinogenic risk to humans from exposure through the diet".*

This is based on available evidence, yet who supplied the evidence and why is it incomplete? Haven't they been using this for close to 40 years. I respectfully, dispute this claim. It is incomplete, in its assessment. Who's withholding the real evidence from them? This makes me wonder, is someone greasing their palms?

Are you glyphosate-resistant? Can your body withstand the changes that glyphosate forces upon your body every time you have a sandwich? With Glyphosate being coated on the corn that your chips are made from, how can you guarantee that none of it is in your body? How can you guarantee that it's not affecting your physiology? Can you guarantee that it's not affecting the actions of enzymes in your body that regulate your health? What guarantees do you have that this won't initiate more trips to your doctor?

Acetylcholine is an important chemical in the body that's important for brain function and muscle function throughout the body as Acetylcholine is a neurotransmitter. For Acetylcholine to act as a neurotransmitter, it needs multiple enzymes that function in the central nervous system and the peripheral nervous system, as Acetylcholine works as a neuromodulator as well as a neurotransmitter.

The body uses the enzyme acetylcholinesterase to help activate muscles by inhibiting the action of **acetylcholine**, and if glyphosate herbicides (Roundup weed killer used on more farms than any other weed killer) are enzyme inhibitors, how can the ingestion of grains laden with these herbicides, not affect the function of the enzymes in your body since you consume them every time you eat bread products of any sort?

According to Wikipedia; *"Acetylcholine receptor agonists and antagonists can either have an effect directly on the receptors or exert their effects indirectly, e.g., by affecting the enzyme acetylcholinesterase (AChE), which degrades the receptor ligand.*

Agonists increase the level of receptor activation, antagonists reduce it."

These Glyphosate herbicides are enzyme inhibitors that have the ability to alter or stop the cell signaling capabilities of enzymes. If they can do this to plants, where is the guarantee that it won't affect your body? Chances are, they're going to change how your body operates and in the long run be the precursor to many diseases. It's crucial for the body's proper function that the actions of certain enzymes are never altered. Where's the guarantee that these enzyme-inhibiting herbicides that your corn, wheat, and potatoes, have been sprayed with, won't affect your enzymatic function, and health? There is none.

In a report from PubMed.com, dated January, 2012;

- **Glyphosate as an acetylcholinesterase inhibitor in Cnesterodon decemmaculatus.**

    "...a significant inhibitory effect on AChE activity was recorded even for the lowest herbicide concentration tested (1 mg L(-1)), in the homogenates corresponding to the anterior body section. The inhibition ranged from 23 to 36%. The analytical determination of glyphosate in assay media by ion chromatography, was used to verify its stability. These results indicate that AChE-a neurotoxicity biomarker-in C. decemmaculatus may be affected by exposure to environmentally relevant concentrations of glyphosate."

It's a little clearer to see now, how, the altering of how enzymes work in our bodies, can have an effect on our health. I can see how this could come from a diet high in grains because of how much of Roundup is sprayed on grain that's milled into flour. I can also see how this could present a huge gain for the pharmaceutical industry. This gives the phrase "cash crop" a whole new meaning.

Is this really the intent of Monsanto? Or is it just negligence? I have to wonder because of their previous ties with Pharmacia & Upjohn, makers of Celebrex. Because of their previous entanglements with other corporations and the law, I'm forced to wonder about their motivations. That is something for you to decide, are they innocent of genocide, or guilty?

I for one would not like to have this inhibitor flowing through by blood mucking up my system. Who knows what enzymes it's going to inhibit in your body? Fortunately for me, I don't have to worry about that, as carbs aren't in my diet. They don't get a chance to muck up anything in my body anymore, I've gone keto and I'm not going back.

It looks to me like Monsanto is trying to lock up not only our digestive problems but the resolve of those digestive problems. They like, to persuade you to buy their food products, which you are more than happy to do, then they get your money again when you purchase your Celebrex to ease the pain of the arthritis given you by their grains.

It's not only Monsanto, Bayer has its own interest in the area of crop science, as explained by Wikipedia, *"in 2002, Bayer AG acquired the Dutch seed company Nunhems, which at the time was one of the world's top five seed companies. In 2006, the U.S. Department of Agriculture announced that Bayer CropScience's Liberty Link genetically modified rice had contaminated the U.S. rice supply. Shortly after the public learned of the contamination, the E.U. banned imports of U.S. long-grain rice and the futures price plunged. In April 2010, a Lonoke County, Arkansas jury awarded a dozen farmers $48 million. The case is currently on appeal to the Arkansas Supreme Court. On 1 July 2011 Bayer CropScience* *agreed to a global settlement for up to $750 million. In September 2014, the firm announced plans to invest $1 billion in the United States between 2013 and 2016. A Bayer spokesperson said that the largest investments will be made to expand the production of its herbicide Liberty. Liberty is used to kill weeds which have grown resistant to Monsanto's product Roundup. I can't help but wonder, what do these chemicals do to the body? How do they kill weeds? Do they also kill humans? I used to wonder about this, but, no more.*

Bayer's involvement

Bayer's four divisions, are related in their concerns to their contribution to our food industry as well as their contribution to the pharmaceutical industry. Bayer Pharmaceuticals, Bayer Crop Science, Bayer Animal Health, and Bayer Consumer Health are all related to our health. They too, like to charge us for the food they market to us, then charge us for medication to treat the symptoms of the diseases that their foods are responsible for. Their divested interests are Lanxess (Bayer Chemicals AG) Diagnostics Division, Diabetes Devices Division, Covestro (Bayer Material Science). With all this influence in your health, how much of their chemicals are you going to allow to influence it?

Astra Zenica / Syngenta's *involvement*

*"Zeneca Agrochemicals was part of **AstraZeneca**, and formerly of **Imperial Chemical Industries**. ICI was formed in the UK in 1926. Two years later, work began at the Agricultural Research Station at **Jealotts Hill** near **Bracknell**." "In 2004, Syngenta Seeds purchased **Garst**, the North American corn and soybean business of Advanta, as well as **Golden Harvest Seeds**. On 5 December 2004, the European Union ended a six-year moratorium when it approved imports of two varieties of **genetically modified corn** sold by Monsanto and its Swiss rival, Syngenta."*

AstraZeneca owned by Syngenta again is evidence of this industrial control over our lives. Syngenta is a Swiss biotechnology company that operates globally. According to Wikipedia; *"Syngenta AG is a global Swiss **agribusiness** that* *produces **agrochemicals** and seeds. As a biotechnology company, it conducts genomic research. It was formed in 2000 by the merger of **Novartis** Agribusiness and **Zeneca** Agrochemicals. As of 2014, Syngenta was the world's largest crop chemical producer, strongest in Europe. As of 2009, it ranked third in seeds and biotechnology sales. Sales in 2015 were approximately US$13.4 billion, over half of which were in **emerging markets**.*"

The three agrichemical companies above are the largest in the world, controlling a majority of the foods we eat along with the medications we take. I'll lay out the evidence of what their foods do to the human body, in the next chapter, because they continue to produce the seed for the crops to make the food they want us to put on our table to eat and you need to know, what you're eating. They also produce the aspirin everybody takes for the headaches they get from eating their bread, and the baby aspirin to keep arteries clean of the plaque created by the glucose. What they won't tell you, is what this does to your kidneys and liver and how it increases the risk of gastrointestinal bleeding. That's alright, though, they make medicine for that, too.

I've said before, how convenient we've made it, for this industry to take our money while slowly, agonizingly, painfully killing us, with their food. But our money is not the only thing they rob us of. They rob us of our dignity as well, for their food does more than anything else, to rob us of our memories. We allow them to do this because of our addiction and none of their foods require warning labels, like that of cigarettes. We also allow it to happen, because of what it does to our brains to knock out our memory and judgment.

We've given this industry our lives and souls by bending to their advertising and buying into their game. We allow them to addict us when we're infants by dumping sugar and corn syrup solids into the baby food we feed our kids. Then we allow them to continue their assault by buying into advertising schemes every Saturday morning with their cereal commercials. To fully hook us they add sugar to this already sugar-laden food simply to make it more palatable.

When an industry does this, how are we supposed to fight the addiction? This makes every American who buys into this behavior a slave to this industry. Slaves make the best captive audience. They have no choice in what they do except to choose their device of demise, Wheaties or cornflakes. If, you put soy milk over either of these, you're eating three of the most heavily glyphosated foods, this industry can sell you. How quick do you think, that could make you sick?

What more do you need, than a captive audience to sell your wares, to? This is why a Coke at a ballgame costs 3 times more than what you can get it for, at the grocery store. At the ballgame, you're a captive audience. It's the same when you're addicted. Every *'PUSHER'* knows this and they charge a premium price for it. They also give you a discounted price, up-front to buy your addiction. This is exactly why everyone who remains in this trap, stays a slave to it, captive to the whims of these industries. *"If you can't afford your medication, AstraZeneca may be able to help you."*

The Litigation Game

These industries are tied up with lawsuits in other areas of their agrichemical businesses. For example, Monsanto has fought legal claims of false advertising, as explained again in Wikipedia;

- *"In 1996, the New York Times reported that: "Dennis C. Vacco, the Attorney General of New York, ordered the company to pull ads that said Roundup was "safer than table salt" and "practically nontoxic" to mammals, birds, and fish. The company withdrew the spots, but also said that the phrase in question was permissible under E.P.A. guidelines."*
- *"In 1999, Monsanto was condemned by the UK Advertising Standards Authority (ASA) for making "confusing, misleading, unproven and wrong" claims about its products over the course of a £1 million advertising campaign. The ASA ruled that Monsanto had presented its opinions "as accepted fact" and had published "wrong" and "unproven"*

scientific claims. Monsanto responded with an apology and claimed it was not intending to deceive and instead "did not take sufficiently into account the difference in culture between the UK and the USA in the way some of this information was presented."

I've not heard better spin from anybody. An LP doesn't spin like that. I'm beginning to think, they must have wrote the book on spin. With their court docket, I wouldn't doubt it.

- *"In 2001, French environmental and consumer rights campaigners brought a case against Monsanto for misleading the public about the environmental impact of its herbicide Roundup, on the basis that glyphosate, Roundup's main ingredient, is classed as "dangerous for the environment" and "toxic for aquatic organisms" by the European Union. Monsanto's advertising for Roundup had presented it as biodegradable and as leaving the soil clean after use. In 2007, Monsanto was convicted of false advertising and was fined 15,000 Euros. Monsanto's French distributor Scotts France was also fined 15,000 Euros. Both defendants were ordered to pay damages of 5,000 Euros to the Brittany Water and Rivers Association and 3,000 Euros to the CLCV (Consommation Logement Cadre de vie), one of the two main general consumer associations in France. Monsanto appealed and the court upheld the verdict; Monsanto appealed again to the French Supreme Court, and in 2009 it also upheld the verdict."*
- *"In August 2012, a Brazilian Regional Federal Court ordered Monsanto to pay a $250,000 fine for false advertising. In 2004, advertising that related to the use of GM soya seed, and the herbicide glyphosate used in its cultivation, claimed it was beneficial to the conservation of the environment. The federal prosecutor maintained that Monsanto misrepresented the amount of herbicide required and stated that "there is no scientific certainty that soybeans marketed by Monsanto use less herbicide." The presiding judge condemned Monsanto and called the advertisement "abusive and misleading propaganda." The prosecutor held that the goal of the advertising was to prepare the market for the purchase of genetically modified soybean seed (sale of which was then banned) and the herbicide used on it, at a time when the approval of a*

- *Brazilian Biosafety Law, enacted in 2005, was being discussed in the country."*
- *"In March 2014 the South African Advertising Standards Authority (ASA) upheld a complaint, made by the African Centre for Biosafety, that Monsanto had made "unsubstantiated" claims about genetically modified crops in its radio advertisements, and ordered that these adverts be pulled. In March 2015 after considering further documentation from Monsanto, the ASA reversed its ruling."*
- *"In 2009, Monsanto came under scrutiny from the U.S. Department of Justice, which began investigating whether the company's activities in the soybean markets were breaking anti-trust rules. In 2010, the Department of Justice created a website through which comments on "Agriculture and Antitrust Enforcement Issues in Our 21st Century Economy" could be submitted; over 15,000 comments were submitted including a letter by 14 State Attorneys General. The comments are publicly available. On November 16, 2012, Monsanto announced that it had received written notification from the U.S. Department of Justice that the Antitrust Division had concluded its inquiry and that the Department of Justice had closed the inquiry without taking any enforcement action. Opponents of Monsanto's seed patenting and licensing practices expressed frustration that the Department of Justice released no information about the results of the inquiry."*
- All of these cases are a clear indication of the extent to which Monsanto is willing to push the limits. This is how corporate risk/loss assessment works. Sometimes the risk of paying a $150,000 find is worth the theft of a patent. My problem with this is they're playing with my health, if I decide to eat their products. So, what are their products? Who knows? Who knows who grows the crops for the corn flakes that you ate this morning for breakfast. Do you? I don't. But I now know it was one of these companies.

Syngenta as well has been accused of making false claims about being involved in suits for false patent infringement.

- *"In 2001, the United States Patent and Trademark Office ruled in favor of Syngenta which had filed a suit against Bayer for patent infringement on a class of neonicotinoid insecticides. The following year Syngenta filed suits against Monsanto and other companies claiming infringement of its U.S. biotechnology patents covering genetically modified corn and cotton. In 2004, it again filed a suit against Monsanto, claiming antitrust violations related to the U.S. biotech corn seed market, and Monsanto countersued. Monsanto and Syngenta settled all litigation in 2008."*

I mention this to point out the extent of their influence in the crop seed industry, where they have 15 of their own seed companies that all provide GMO crop seed for farmers to plant for their crops for food which ends up on our tables. Syngenta is the second largest chemical corporation in the industry, Monsanto is even larger. And when we considered Bayer CropScience, DOW AgroSciences or DuPont Pioneer, we're considering 97% of the food provided for our tables.

Most of these cases involve patent rights to GMO seed with companies like Monsanto or DuPont Pioneer. It's not just patent problems; most of these companies like to make out that their products are completely harmless to the environment when they've been proven otherwise.

- *"Syngenta was a defendant in a class action lawsuit by the city of Greenville, Illinois concerning the adverse effects of atrazine in human water supplies. The suit was settled for $105 million in May 2012. A similar case involving six states has been in federal court since 2010."*
- *"In the US, Syngenta is facing lawsuits from farmers and shipping companies regarding Viptera genetically modified corn. The plaintiffs in nearly 30 states contend that Syngenta's introduction of Viptera drove down US grain market prices, leading to financial harm and that Syngenta acted irresponsibly by doing too little to enable shipping companies to export the grain to approved ports. Before Vipera's 2010 introduction*

Syngenta secured all US and NCGA-recommended export approvals, but none from China. China had imported little to no US grain prior to 2010, and at the time was not considered a major partner, but it became a major partner in 2010 when it dramatically increased US grain imports. For three years, China imported U.S. Viptera grain without formal approval. In November 2013, Chinese officials destroyed a U.S. grain shipment containing Viptera grain, started rejecting all US shipments with the GM grain, but continued to accept it from all countries other than the US. That same year, US corn market prices dropped $4 per bushel, causing over $2.9B in losses, with just over half of that loss occurring prior to China's November rejection. China later approved the GM corn in 2014 but US corn grain market prices have not rebounded."

The choice is yours

These are the kind of companies that are ultimately providing your food. Do you want them making your drugs also? As you've seen, they already do. Do you wonder why the prevalence of these diseases is so rampant? It's in these industries' best interest that this cycle continues.

We've allowed this to take place, right under our noses and we should be ashamed. Doesn't this sound a lot like a wicked witch luring small children with candy and sweets? Because of our addiction, we continue this behavior.

This addiction has and is costing America more money and lives than any other addiction that we've ever experienced. There are 48,000,000 deaths worldwide each year due to ECC, excessive carbohydrate consumption. There were 17.3 million deaths in 2013 alone due to cardiovascular disease. Cancer claims over 4 million each year and Alzheimer's disease takes 5 million each year, yet I hear no outrage about it. All of these deaths and suffering can be curbed simply by curbing carbohydrate consumption. It's time to put an end to this addiction. It's time for a cure. But to stop the addiction, you first have to **De-Celebratize** it. We have to stop celebrating its addictive qualities and exchange that celebration, for castigation of the horror, for what, this addiction really does.

Everybody needs to think about what harm this food does before they put it in their mouth instead of thinking how good it tastes. Unfortunately for my generation and all those that have come along since, we're stuck in the quicksand of addiction that we have to carry with us for the rest of our lives. Even most natural causes of death happen, in part, due to what this food has done to the body over the lifetime of the deceased. An autopsy will likely show some form of arthritis, as this is evidence of the inflammation, oxidative stress and cell degradation that these foods cause. If the inflammation, oxidative stress and cell degradation exists in the joints, it has to exist elsewhere in the body and since it exists throughout the body, as that's where inflammation exists, in the blood. So, it has to affect everything it comes in contact with. That means it affects your heart, your brain, and every internal organ. How can that not have an effect on your life? It has to, so I have to ask, why is this food still allowed to be sold without a warning about just how dangerous it is? Cigarettes require one. Alcohol does. Heroin is illegal and opioids require prescriptions. But not the one substance that minimizes all the damage caused by these other substances collectively, sugar from grains requires no warning of the damage it inflicts. Why?

Going back to the problems this industry has had in court, mostly protecting their patents and falsely claiming that their products are harmless when they're not. Most of the patent problems lie in the resistance their new crop seeds have to their insecticides and pesticides, which have proven to have effects in the human body. Yet they are still allowed to spray their crops with these herbicides and pesticides. My question is, how much of these herbicides and pesticides trickle into our food supply? How confident are you that no chemicals are in what you eat? How confident are you that no enzyme controlling chemicals are not in your biscuits or crackers? How confident are you that your sugar addiction won't turn into diabetes? How confident are you that your addiction won't turn into heart disease or cancer? Whether you worry about it or not, you will experience brain loss. That's just in the science. You can't change it without saying goodbye to your addiction. This obviously isn't easy with a grain industry that feeds the pharmaceutical industry. I'm sorry that this industry seems to have no intention of changing that and helping you out.

THE DANGER IN GLYCTION

LIES IN THE ACCUMULATION

OF ALL THE INFLAMMATION

RAMPED UP BY GLYPHOSATION

FORCING YOU TO TAKE MORE MEDICATION

TO QUELL YOUR PAINFUL OBLIGATION

BROUGHT ON BY YOUR CELEBRATION

IT'S TIME TO SAY NO TO THE INDUSTRY THAT FEEDS YOU,

SO YOU CAN SAY NO TO THE INDUSTRY THAT DRUGS YOU.

LEARN TO 'JUST SAY NO' TO GRAINS AND DRUGS

IT'S IN YOUR INTEREST TO KEEP YOUR RUG

SO YOUR HEALTH YOU WON'T HAVE TO SHRUG

TO SATISFY YOUR ADDICTION TO THIS DRUG,

SUGAR

IV

The Dangers of Glycation

As much as I love vegans and vegetarianism, it's become too much of a carb intense diet for my body. My cholesterol is too high to take in any carbs. With that said, I used to be a vegetarian, and I actually lost weight the first time I went vegan, which was quite a while ago. I think the weight I lost was due to loss of muscle tissue, which is heavier than fat.

I've learned since quitting bread, how much damage carbs really do, to the body. I won't touch them ever again. They're just too dangerous, especially since I now live with higher cholesterol. I learned that higher cholesterol has made me more intelligent than I was when I was on a carb diet. That's another myth that the food industry wants you to think, that high cholesterol is dangerous and leads to disease. Cholesterol may be in the equation, but it's not the instigator. Carbs are.

It's the glycation factor that makes carbs so bad. Only carbs can cause glycation, nothing else. Only carbs can create high blood pressure. Only carbs can create heart disease and cancer. Only carbs create the inflammation that's necessary to initiate these diseases. Keep in mind that it's the insulin that really adds the fat. It's when this hormone runs out, the glycation kicks up exponentially, to escalate glycations' destruction. That's what makes diabetes so deadly and the doorway to all other diseases. This is the inherent danger of a carb diet or a vegetarian diet. That risk doesn't exist with a ketogenic diet of any sort. No one on a ketogenic diet has become diabetic, since carbs are just a very small part of a ketogenic diet, the glycation factor is next to negligible for those in ketosis. It comes gift wrapped with all carb diets, which gives you the gift of glycation. If, you're looking for glycation, carbs will give you, as much as you want. My question, who wants it? What follows shows you why, I don't, won't, and can't.

The Real Poisoning of America - Glycation

According to PubMed article;

- **"Potentially preventable deaths from the five leading causes of death--United States, 2008-2010.figures"**

"In 2010, the top five causes of death in the United States were 1) diseases of the heart, 2) cancer, 3) chronic lower respiratory diseases, 4) cerebrovascular diseases (stroke), and 5) unintentional injuries. The rates of death from each cause vary greatly across the 50 states and the District of Columbia (2). An understanding of state differences in death rates for the leading causes might help state health officials establish disease prevention goals, priorities, and strategies. States with lower death rates can be used as benchmarks for setting achievable goals and calculating the number of deaths that might be prevented in states with higher rates. To determine the number of premature annual deaths for the five leading causes of death that potentially could be prevented ("potentially preventable deaths"), CDC analyzed National Vital Statistics System mortality data from 2008-2010. The number of annual potentially preventable deaths per state before age 80 years was determined by comparing the number of expected deaths (based on average death rates for the three states with the lowest rates for each cause) with the number of observed deaths. The results of this analysis indicate that, when considered separately, 91,757 deaths from diseases of the heart, 84,443 from cancer, 28,831 from chronic lower respiratory diseases, 16,973 from cerebrovascular diseases (stroke), and 36,836 from unintentional injuries potentially could be prevented each year. In addition, states in the Southeast had the highest number of potentially preventable deaths for each of the five leading causes. The findings provide disease-specific targets that states can use to measure their progress in preventing the leading causes of deaths in their populations."

Figures are hard to find for recent years, as a lot of causes are age related. The older a person gets, the greater his chances of dying of ECC. Cancer, though attacks even babies, but historically takes people over 40. Heart disease and cardiovascular diseases combined, make for the number one killer of your neighbors and friends. 89% of preventable deaths or 20 million are directly linked to ECC, Excessive Carbohydrate Consumption, making them the most preventable causes of death. 20 million deaths each and every year amounts to over 54,794 people every day. That includes approximately 2191 Americans each and every day. We have full control of this. All it would take is to say no to the sugar and grain industries. This one response would allow over 2191 more Americans to stay alive, every day. The cessation of carb consumption could add an additional 10-20 years to their lives, simply by eliminating the primary cause of inflammation, glucose. The continuation of carb consumption will, by contrast, prove the destructive power of sugar, by eventually killing its hosts.

Glycation is a common everyday experience that you accelerate with a carbohydrate diet. The more carbs you eat, the more glycation you'll get to deal with. Glycation is controllable by controlling what you put in your mouth to eat. Although not totally responsible for some of these cancers, they would not exist if the glycation didn't exist. This is the basis of my contention that if you eliminate the reason for the glycation, you eliminate the reason for inflammation, which in turn will eliminate the reason for these diseases, thereby eliminating the disease. It's really not hard to see, once you take a good look at it; carb consumption is responsible for the inflammation that builds in the blood that is responsible for 89% of all modern diseases. Remove the inflammation by removing the sugar, which means removing the carbs. A simpler solution doesn't exist and this cure can be yours.

For the following reports, clarifications to these acronyms will help to understand what's being expressed in the bulk of these studies;

1. age; *advanced glycation end-product*

2. rage: *receptor for advanced glycation end-product*

3. srage: *soluble receptor for advanced glycation end-product*:

4. esrage: *endogenous secretory receptor for advanced glycation-end products*

5. You'll find other acronyms, such as HMGB-1; *This gene encodes a protein that belongs to the High Mobility Group-box superfamily. The encoded non-histone, nuclear DNA-binding protein regulates transcription and is involved in organization of DNA. This protein plays a role in several cellular processes, including inflammation, cell differentiation and tumor cell migration.*

*These are the smoking gun, articles
of evidence that the FDA are ignoring.
In doing so, they're putting your health and life at risk.*

Around 50 of the 23,551 studies done on glycation are below. These research studies were chosen from 231 studies that I examined for evidence of what glycation does to the body. By going through only 7% of these studies, I was able to find enough damning evidence to condemn this food 31 times over. By this ratio, I'll end up finding at the least 850 more studies showing damage that glycation does.

I chose to search glycation because I know that it's at the root of all modern diseases from cancer to CVDs to arthritis to dementia including Alzheimer disease. The following studies are the proof of what glycation does, and with sugar being the primary instigator of glycation, removal of sugar from the diet will eliminate everything it's responsible for.

The study that piqued my interest initially was the report on RAGEs; This report can be found at PubMed.gov. It explains how glycation turns your body's fuel into AGEs before it can be used for fuel. These AGEs are responsible for all modern diseases and thus, are the reason for this chapter.

- **_Receptor for advanced glycation end-products-mediated inflammation and diabetic vascular complications._**
"Exposure of amino residue of proteins to reducing sugars, such as glucose, glucose 6-phosphate, fructose, ribose and intermediate aldehydes, results in non-enzymatic glycation, which forms reversible schiff bases and amadori compounds. A series of further complex molecular rearrangements then yield irreversible advanced glycation end-products (age). The aldehydes, highly reactive age precursors, are produced by both enzymatic and non-enzymatic pathways. The enzymatic pathways include a route of myeloperoxidase in inflammatory cells, such as activated macrophages, which produces hypochlorite, then reacting with serine to generate glycolaldehyde." Is this something you want mucking up your body?
Here's a good explanation of glycation and how it works and what it affects, as this shows evidence of glycation's involvement in all neurodegenerative diseases, including Alzheimer's disease, Parkinson's disease and Huntington's disease from Nov 18, 2016

- **_Glycation potentiates neurodegeneration in models of Huntington's disease_**

    "Glucose is the major energy supply of neurons and is essential for their survival. However, impaired glucose metabolism can also damage neurons and lead to neurodegeneration. For example, diabetic patients who neglect their circulating glucose levels frequently develop severe neuropathy that results in the amputation of limbs. Glucose metabolism drives the formation of by-products that are highly reactive with free amino-groups of proteins. This non-enzymatic reaction, named glycation, induces the formation of advanced glycation end-products (AGEs) that frequently have deleterious effects on proteins. For example, glycation has been reported in several neurodegenerative disorders such as Alzheimer's and Parkinson's diseases, where it potentiates the aggregation and toxicity of proteins such as amyloid-β (Aβ) and α-synuclein, respectively."

I wonder if this last study, completed a few years ago, is publicized in the media for the AMA, ADA, or even FDA yet. I have my doubts. I wonder when it will be. At the present rate of informing the public of what eating this food entails, it won't ever be publicized. Do you think this is something that is important enough that everyone should know it? Have you heard about any preventative cure for any of these diseases? You've only heard about using insulin to fix this problem of excess glucose. Insulin adds fat. Has your doctor ever shared anything of this nature, with you? Does (s)he know? Would he care, if he did? Or, does he appreciate, more, your return visits, from being fat and diabetic? Can't your doctor learn that a patient that lives longer and healthier will ultimately keep him in business, longer?

The following report is the evidence of glucose's involvement in arthritis. By being responsible for glycation, the glucose from broken down carbs, again, is directly responsible for arthritis

- **_"PROTEIN OXIDATION, NITRATION AND GLYCATION BIOMARKERS FOR EARLY-STAGE DIAGNOSIS OF OSTEOARTHRITIS OF THE KNEE AND TYPING AND PROGRESSION OF ARTHRITIC DISEASE."_**

    "Glycated, oxidized and nitrated proteins and amino acids were detected in synovial fluid and plasma of arthritic patients with characteristic patterns found in early and advanced oa and ra, and non-ra, with respect to healthy controls. In early-stage disease, two

algorithms for consecutive use in diagnosis were developed: (1) disease versus healthy control, and (2) classification as oa, ra and non-ra."

The following report show the effects that AGEs have on the body in the diseases it promotes.

- **"EFFECT OF GLYCATION INHIBITORS ON AGING AND AGE-RELATED DISEASES."**

"Vast evidence supports the view that glycation of proteins is one of the main factors contributing to aging and is an important element of etiopathology of age-related diseases, especially type 2 diabetes mellitus, cataract, and neurodegenerative diseases.
Counteracting glycation can, therefore, be a means of increasing both the lifespan and health span. In this review, accumulation of glycation products during aging is presented, pathophysiological effects of glycation are discussed and ways of attenuation of the effects of glycation are described, concentrating on prevention of glycation. The effects of glycation and glycation inhibitors on the course of selected age-related diseases, such as alzheimer's disease, parkinson's disease, and cataract are also reviewed."

I have to ask myself, would these "age-related" diseases exist if glycation didn't? How long could that extend our lifespan?

This study looks at the damaging effects of glycation along with the protective effects of certain phytochemicals (anti-oxidant producing agents).

- **"PHYTOCHEMICALS AGAINST ADVANCED GLYCATION END PRODUCTS (AGES) AND THE RECEPTOR SYSTEM."**

"Reducing sugars can react non-enzymatically with amino groups of proteins and lipids to form irreversibly cross-linked macroprotein derivatives called as advanced glycation end products (ages). Cross-linking modification of extracellular matrix proteins by ages deteriorate their tertiary structural integrity and function, contributing to aging-related organ damage and diabetes-associated complications, such as cardiovascular disease (cvd). Moreover, engagement of receptor for ages, rage with the ligands evoke oxidative stress generation and inflammatory, thrombotic and fibrotic reactions in various kinds of tissues, further exacerbating the deleterious effects of ages on multiple organ systems. So the age-rage axis is a novel therapeutic target for numerous devastating

disorders. Several observational studies have shown the association of dietary consumption of fruits and vegetables with the reduced risk of cvd in a general population. Although beneficial effects of fruits and vegetables against cvd could mainly be ascribed to its anti-oxidative properties, blockade of the age-rage axis by phytochemicals may also contribute to cardiovascular event protection. Therefore, in this review, we focus on 4 phytochemicals (quercetin, sulforaphane, iridoids, and curcumin) and summarize their effects on age formation as well as rage-mediated signaling pathway in various cell types and organs, including endothelial cells, vessels, and heart."

This report examines the nature of amyloid plaque and glyoxal (Glyoxal is an **inflammatory** compound formed when **cooking oils** and **fats** are heated to high temperatures). Glyoxal is also part of methylglyoxal and the glyoxalase system which pertains to detoxification of the methylglyoxal and removal of contaminants from the body. To explain how the system works, from Wikipedia:

The glyoxalase system is a set of enzymes that carry out the detoxification of methylglyoxal and the other reactive aldehydes that are produced as a normal part of metabolism. This system has been studied in both bacteria and eukaryotes.

- **"GLYOXAL ADMINISTRATION INDUCES FORMATION OF HIGH MOLECULAR WEIGHT AGGREGATES OF HEMOGLOBIN EXHIBITING AMYLOIDAL NATURE IN EXPERIMENTAL RATS: AN IN VIVO STUDY."**

"Glyoxal, a highly reactive α-oxoaldehyde, increases in diabetic condition and reacts with proteins to form advanced glycation end products (ages). In the present study, we have investigated the effect of glyoxal on experimental rat hemoglobin in vivo after external administration of the α-dicarbonyl compound in animals. Gel electrophoretic profile of hemolysate collected from glyoxal-treated rats (32mg/kg body wt. Dose) after one week exhibited the presence of some high molecular weight protein bands that were found to be absent for control, untreated rats. Mass spectrometric and absorption studies indicated that the bands represented hemoglobin. Further studies revealed that the fraction exhibited the presence of intermolecular cross β-sheet structure. Thus glyoxal administration induces formation of high molecular weight aggregates of hemoglobin with amyloid characteristics in rats. Aggregated hemoglobin fraction was found to exhibit higher stability compared to glyoxal-untreated hemoglobin. As evident from mass spectrometric studies, glyoxal was found to modify arg-30β and arg-31α of rat hemoglobin to hydroimidazolone adducts. The

modifications thus appear to induce amyloid-like aggregation of hemoglobin in rats. Considering the increased level of glyoxal in diabetes mellitus as well as its high reactivity, the above findings may be physiologically significant."

*"In view of its inflammatory function in innate immunity and its ability to detect a class of **ligands** through a common **structural motif**, rage is often referred to as a **pattern recognition receptor.**"*

Methylglyoxal is the link from glucose to disease through its conversion to AGEs, advanced glycation endproducts as explained by this study;

- **"Methylglyoxal in Metabolic Disorders: Facts, Myths, and Promises."**

"Glucose and fructose metabolism originates the highly reactive by-product methylglyoxal (mg), which is a strong precursor of advanced glycation end products (age). The mg has been implicated in classical diabetic complications such as retinopathy, nephropathy, and neuropathy, but has also been recently associated with cardiovascular diseases and central nervous system disorders such as cerebrovascular diseases and dementia. Recent studies even suggested its involvement in insulin resistance and beta-cell dysfunction, contributing to the early development of type 2 diabetes and creating a vicious circle between glycation and hyperglycemia. Despite several drugs and natural compounds have been identified in the last years in order to scavenge mg and inhibit age formation, we are still far from having an effective strategy to prevent mg-induced mechanisms. This review summarizes the endogenous and exogenous sources of mg, also addressing the current controversy about the importance of exogenous mg sources. The mechanisms by which mg changes cell behavior and its involvement in type 2 diabetes development and complications and the pathophysiological implication are also summarized. Particular emphasis will be given to the pathophysiological relevance of studies using higher mg doses, which may have produced biased results. Finally, we also overview the current knowledge about detoxification strategies, including modulation of endogenous enzymatic systems and exogenous compounds able to inhibit mg effects on biological systems."

It seems to me the more carbs a person eats, the more glyoxal they get to deal with. Is this something you've been warned about? I haven't. This following report examines the relationship of high mobility group box 1 (HMGB1) and the effects it has on the body. HMGB1 is quite possibly the most prevalent AGE;

- **"HMGB1 ACTIVATES PROINFLAMMATORY SIGNALING VIA TLR5 LEADING TO ALLODYNIA."**
(Pain that results from a noninjurious stimulus to the skin.)
"Infectious and sterile inflammatory diseases are correlated with increased levels of high mobility group box 1 (hmgb1) in tissues and serum. Extracellular hmgb1 is known to activate toll-like receptors (tlrs) 2 and 4 and rage (receptor for advanced glycation end products) in inflammatory conditions. Here, we find that tlr5 is also an hmgb1 receptor that was previously overlooked due to lack of functional expression in the cell lines usually used for studying tlr signaling. Hmgb1 binding to tlr5 initiates the activation of nf-κb signaling pathway in a myd88-dependent manner, resulting in pro-inflammatory cytokine production and pain enhancement in vivo. Biophysical and in vitro results highlight an essential role for the c-terminal tail region of hmgb1 in facilitating interactions with tlr5. These results suggest that hmgb1-modulated tlr5 signaling is responsible for pain hypersensitivity."

Is this pain hypersensitivity something you would want in your body? This is what drove me to suicide's doorstep. The proof that carb consumption also contributes to COPD is in the following report. The underlying cause is inflammation.

- **"THE SER82 RAGE VARIANT AFFECTS LUNG FUNCTION AND SERUM RAGE IN SMOKERS AND SRAGE PRODUCTION IN VITRO."**
"ABSTRACT"
INTRODUCTION:
Genome-Wide Association Studies have identified associations between lung function measures and Chronic Obstructive Pulmonary Disease (COPD) and chromosome region 6p21 containing the gene for the Advanced Glycation End Product Receptor (AGER, encoding RAGE). We aimed to (i) characterize RAGE expression in the lung, (ii) identify AGER transcripts, (iii) ascertain if SNP rs2070600 (Gly82Ser C/T) is associated with lung function and serum sRAGE levels and (iv) identify whether the Gly82Ser variant is functionally important in altering sRAGE levels in an airway epithelial cell model.
METHODS:
Immunohistochemistry was used to identify RAGE protein expression in 26 human tissues and qPCR was used to quantify AGER mRNA in lung cells. Gene expression array data was used to identify AGER expression during lung development in 38 fetal lung samples. RNA-Seq was used to identify AGER transcripts in lung cells. sRAGE levels were assessed in cells

and patient serum by ELISA. BEAS2B-R1 cells were transfected to overexpress RAGE protein with either the Gly82 or Ser82 variant and sRAGE levels identified.
RESULTS:
Immunohistochemical assessment of 6 adult lung samples identified high RAGE expression in the alveoli of healthy adults and individuals with COPD. AGER/RAGE expression increased across developmental stages in human fetal lung at both the mRNA (38 samples) and protein levels (20 samples). Extensive AGER splicing was identified. The rs2070600T (Ser82) allele is associated with higher FEV1, FEV1/FVC and lower serum sRAGE levels in UK smokers. Using an airway epithelium model overexpressing the Gly82 or Ser82 variants we found that HMGB1 activation of the RAGE-Ser82 receptor results in lower sRAGE production.
CONCLUSIONS:
This study provides new information regarding the expression profile and potential role of RAGE in the human lung and shows a functional role of the Gly82Ser variant. These findings advance our understanding of the potential mechanisms underlying COPD particularly for carriers of this AGER polymorphism."

This begs the question, would lung cancer exist, without the glycation? The glycation requires glucose, to take place. How many questions does that raise? Remember the HMGB-1 I mentioned earlier? It exposes it's ugly nature here also.

- ***"CLINICAL VALUE OF HIGH MOBILITY GROUP BOX 1 AND THE RECEPTOR FOR ADVANCED GLYCATION END-PRODUCTS IN HEAD AND NECK CANCER: A SYSTEMATIC REVIEW."***

"Introduction high mobility group box 1 is a versatile protein involved in gene transcription, extracellular signaling, and response to inflammation. Extracellularly, high mobility group box 1 binds to several receptors, notably the receptor for advanced glycation end-products. Expression of high mobility group box 1 and the receptor for advanced glycation end-products has been described in many cancers.
OBJECTIVES to systematically review the available literature using pubmed and web of science to evaluate the clinical value of high mobility group box 1 and the receptor for
advanced glycation end-products in head and neck squamous cell carcinomas.
DATA SYNTHESIS
A total of eleven studies were included in this review. High mobility group box 1 overexpression is associated with poor prognosis and

many clinical and pathological characteristics of head and neck squamous cell carcinomas patients. Additionally, the receptor for advanced glycation end-products demonstrates potential value as a clinical indicator of tumor angiogenesis and advanced staging. In diagnosis, high mobility group box 1 demonstrates low sensitivity.
CONCLUSION
High mobility group box 1 and the receptor for advanced glycation end-products are associated with clinical and pathological characteristics of head and neck squamous cell carcinomas. Further investigation of the prognostic and diagnostic value of these molecules is warranted."

This study shows glycation's implication in cardiovascular disease and in my opinion, cannot be understated. I've lost 4 family members to heart disease;

- **"THERAPEUTIC INTERVENTIONS FOR ADVANCED GLYCATION-END PRODUCTS AND ITS RECEPTOR-MEDIATED CARDIOVASCULAR DISEASE."**

"Advanced glycation end products (ages) are a heterogeneous group of molecules formed from non-enzymatic reaction of reducing sugars with amino group of proteins, lipids, and nucleic acid. Interaction of ages with its cell-bound receptor (rage) results in generation of oxygen radicals, nuclear factor kappa-β, pro-inflammatory cytokines and cell adhesion molecules, and is involved in the pathophysiology of cardiovascular diseases (cvd). Circulating soluble forms of rage (srage) and endo-secretory rage (esrage) compete with rage for ligand binding and function as a decoy. This paper describes the endogenous and exogenous (high dietary ages, cooking food under high dry heat, elevated ph, and long period) sources of ages. Age-rage-mediated cvd includes atherosclerosis, coronary artery disease, carotid artery disease, hypertension, peripheral vascular diseases, heart failure, cardiomyopathy, and microangiopathy. The therapeutic intervention with reduction in ages and rage and elevation in srage has been reported for the treatment of age-rage-mediated cvd. Reduction in levels of ages can be achieved by a reduction in consumption of food containing a low amount of ages, cooking food at low temperature, moist heat, and shorter duration. Age formation can be reduced with drugs, vitamins, and stoppage of cigarette smoking. Statins, telmisartan, and curcumin have been used for suppression of rage. Statins, ace-inhibitors, rosiglitazone and vitamin d have been used to increase levels of srage. Finally, exogenous administration of srage can be helpful in amelioration of cvd. In conclusion, age-rage-mediated cvd could be attenuated with a reduction in consumption of ages,

suppression of rage and elevation of srage." Did you see that last line? 'Reduction in consumption of ages'. How do you do that? There's only one way, and that's to stop the glycation, by removing the glucose. That just means to curb your carbs.

How many family members have you lost to cvd's and heart disease? Were any of your family warned about this? Mine wasn't and that's why so many in my family have died from this.
This is evidence of glycation's effect on the kidneys:

- **"AGES/SRAGE, A NOVEL RISK FACTOR IN THE PATHOGENESIS OF END-STAGE RENAL DISEASE."**

"Interaction of advanced glycation end products (ages) with its cell-bound receptor (rage) results in cell dysfunction through activation of nuclear factor kappa-b, increase in expression and release of inflammatory cytokines, and generation of oxygen radicals. Circulating soluble receptors, soluble receptor (srage), endogenous secretory receptor (esrage) and cleaved receptor (crgae) act as a decoy for rage ligands and thus have cytoprotective effects. Low levels of srage and esrage have been proposed as biomarkers for many diseases. However, srage and esrage levels are elevated in diabetes and chronic renal diseases and still tissue injury occurs. It is possible that increases in levels of ages are greater than increases in the levels of soluble receptors in these two diseases. Some new parameters have to be used which could be a universal biomarker for cell dysfunction. It is hypothesized that increases in serum levels of ages are greater than the increases in the soluble receptors, and that the levels of ages is correlated with soluble receptors and that the ratios of ages/srage, ages/esrage, and ages/crage are elevated in patients with end-stage renal disease (esrd) and would serve as a universal risk marker for esrd. The study subject comprised of 88 patients with esrd and 20 healthy controls. Ages, srage, and esrage were measured using commercially available enzyme-linked immune assay kits. Crage was calculated by subtracting esrage from srage. The data show that the serum levels of ages, srage, crage are elevated and that the elevation of ages was greater than those of soluble receptors. The ratios of ages/srage, ages/esrage and ages/crage were elevated and the elevation was similar in ages/srage and ages/crage but greater than ages/esrage. The sensitivity, specificity, accuracy, and positive and negative predictive value of ages/srage and ages/crage were 86.36 and 84.88 %, 86.36 and 80.95 %, 0.98 and 0.905, 96.2 and 94.8 %, and 61.29 and 56.67 % respectively. There was a positive correlation of srage with esrage and crage, and ages with esrage; and a negative correlation between srage and ages/srage,

esrage and ages/esrage, and crage and ages/crage. In conclusion, ages/srage, ages/crage, and ages/esrage may serve as universal risk biomarkers for esrd and that ages/srage and ages/crage are better risk biomarkers than ages/esrage."

This report prompts questions in my mind, What would happen in your body if these ages, rages, srages, esrages, crages didn't exist in the first place, or didn't have to? Wouldn't your life be better off, without the inflammation they create and regulate? Keep in mind that a lot of kidney problems arise from the abundant use of NSAIDs and painkillers.

This is the evidence that breast cancer is influenced by glycation. It's what took my mother. My aunt lost two breasts from her bout with it;

- **"INCREASED EXPRESSION OF THE RECEPTOR FOR ADVANCED GLYCATION END-PRODUCTS (RAGE) IS ASSOCIATED WITH ADVANCED BREAST CANCER STAGE."**

"ABSTRACT"

BACKGROUND:
The receptor for advanced glycation end-products (rage) is a multiligand transmembrane receptor that is overexpressed in various pathological conditions including cancers. However, the expression pattern of rage in breast cancer tumors is still not completely clear.

METHODS:
In this study, we investigated the expression levels of rage in 25 fresh-frozen breast cancer samples and corresponding noncancerous tissue samples collected from breast cancer patients, by real-time polymerase chain reaction (pcr). Additionally, we performed immunohistochemistry on breast cancer specimens.

RESULTS:
the results indicate a high expression of the rage-encoding gene in the cancerous tissues. rage expression at the mrna and protein levels was statistically significantly up-regulated in advanced-stage and triple-negative breast tumors and node-positive tissues compared with other tissues ($p < 0.001$). a significant association between rage expression and tumor size was observed ($p = 0.029$).

CONCLUSIONS:
Overexpression of rage in advanced-stage tumors may be a useful biomarker for diagnosis and the prediction of breast cancer progression."

This evidence of bone density decline from glycation is the start of osteoporosis;

- ***"ADVANCED GLYCATION END PRODUCTS, DIABETES, AND BONE STRENGTH."***

"Diabetic patients have a higher fracture risk than expected by their bone mineral density (bmd). Poor bone quality is the most suitable and explainable cause for the elevated fracture risk in this population. Advanced glycation end products (ages), which are diverse compounds generated via a non-enzymatic reaction between reducing sugars and amine residues, physically affect the properties of the bone material, one of a component of bone quality, through their accumulation in the bone collagen fibers. On the other hand, these compounds biologically act as agonists for these receptors for ages (rage) and suppress bone metabolism. The concentrations of ages and endogenous secretory rage, which acts as a "decoy receptor" that inhibits the ages-rage signaling axis, are associated with fracture risk in a bmd-independent manner. Ages are closely associated with the pathogenesis of this unique clinical manifestation through physical and biological mechanisms in patients with diabetes mellitus."

Evidence of Alzheimer's disease from glycation;
- ***"GENETIC ASSOCIATION BETWEEN RAGE POLYMORPHISMS AND ALZHEIMER'S DISEASE AND LEWY BODY DEMENTIAS IN A** Japanese cohort: a case-control study."*

"ABSTRACT"
BACKGROUND/AIMS:
Interaction of receptor for advanced glycation end products (rage) with amyloid-β increases amplification of oxidative stress and plays pathological roles in alzheimer's disease (ad). Oxidative stress leads to α-synuclein aggregation and is also a major contributing factor in the pathogenesis of lewy body dementias (lbds). Therefore, we aimed to investigate whether rage gene polymorphisms were associated with ad and lbds.
METHODS:
Four single nucleotide polymorphisms (snps)-rs1800624, rs1800625, rs184003, and rs2070600-of the gene were analyzed using a case-control study design comprising 288 ad patients, 76 lbds patients, and 105 age-matched controls.
RESULTS:
Linkage disequilibrium (ld) examination showed strong ld from rs1800624 to rs2070600 on the gene (1.1 kb) in our cases in japan.

Rs184003 was associated with an increased risk of ad. Although there were no statistical associations for the other three snps, haplotypic analyses detected genetic associations between ad and the rage gene. Although relatively few cases were studied, results from the snps showed that they did not modify the risk of developing lbds in the japanese population.
CONCLUSION:
Our findings suggested that polymorphisms in the rage gene are involved in genetic susceptibility to ad. Copyright © 2016 John Wiley & sons, ltd."

More evidence of cancer-causing agents from glycation;

- **"M2 MACROPHAGES DO NOT FLY INTO A "RAGE"."**

"Tumor-associated macrophages (tams) are key elements in orchestrating host responses inside tumor stroma. This population may undergo a polarized activation process, thus rendering a heterogeneous spectrum of phenotypes, where the classically activated type 1 macrophages (m1) and the alternative activated type 2 macrophages (m2) represent two extreme phenotypes. In this commentary, based on very recent research findings, we intend to highlight how complex could be the crosstalk among all components of tumor stroma, where the coexistence of non-natural partners may even skew the canonical responses that we can expect."

Evidence of glycation causing agents in baby food, This is how your addiction is fed, once your born;

- **"PROTEIN BREAKDOWN AND RELEASE OF B-CASOMORPHINS DURING IN VITRO GASTROINTESTINAL DIGESTION OF STERILIZED MODEL SYSTEMS OF LIQUID INFANT FORMULA."**

"Protein modifications occurring during sterilization of infant formulas can affect protein digestibility and release of bioactive peptides. The effect of glycation and cross-linking on protein breakdown and release of β-casomorphins was evaluated during in vitro gastrointestinal digestion (gid) of six sterilized model systems of infant formula. Protein degradation during in vitro gid was evaluated by sds-page and by measuring the nitrogen content of ultrafiltration (3kda) permeates before and after in vitro gid of model ifs. Glycation strongly hindered protein breakdown, whereas cross-linking resulting from β-elimination reactions had a negligible effect. Only β-casomorphin 7 (β-cm7) was detected (0.187-0.858mgl(-1)) at the end of the intestinal digestion in all untreated if model systems. The level of β-cm7 in the sterilized model systems prepared without

addition of sugars ranged from 0.256 to 0.655mgl(-1). The release of this peptide during gid was hindered by protein glycation."

When I looked at the ingredients of Similac baby formula the other day on the grocery shelf, it was 90% corn syrup solids and sugar, thereby stimulating this glycation. Do you still wonder how babies get cancer?

Here's what glucose is responsible for in type 1 diabetics;

- **"THE RECEPTOR FOR ADVANCED GLYCATION ENDPRODUCTS DRIVES T CELL SURVIVAL AND INFLAMMATION IN TYPE 1 DIABETES MELLITUS."**

"The ways in which environmental factors participate in the progression of autoimmune diseases are not known. After initiation, it takes years before hyperglycemia develops in patients at risk for type 1 diabetes (t1d). The receptor for advanced glycation endproducts (rage) is a scavenger receptor of the ig family that binds damage-associated molecular patterns and advanced glycated endproducts and can trigger cell activation. We previously found constitutive intracellular rage expression in lymphocytes from patients with t1d. In this article, we show that there is increased rage expression in t cells from at-risk euglycemic relatives who progress to t1d compared with healthy control subjects, and in the cd8⁺ t cells in the at-risk relatives who do versus those who do not progress to t1d. Detectable levels of the rage ligand high mobility group box 1 were present in serum from at-risk subjects and patients with t1d. Transcriptome analysis of rage⁺ versus rage⁻ t cells from patients with t1d showed differences in signaling pathways associated with increased cell activation and survival. Additional markers for effector memory cells and inflammatory function were elevated in the rage⁺ cd8⁺ cells of t1d patients and at-risk relatives of patients before disease onset. These studies suggest that expression of rage in t cells of subjects progressing to disease predates dysglycemia. These findings imply that rage expression enhances the inflammatory function of t cells, and its increased levels observed in t1d patients may account for the chronic autoimmune response when damage-associated molecular patterns are released after cell injury and killing."

Evidence of the role of AGEs in the process of aging (wrinkling skin, graying hair);

- **"IMPACT OF NON-ENZYMATIC GLYCATION IN NEURODEGENERATIVE DISEASES: ROLE OF NATURAL PRODUCTS IN PREVENTION."**

    "Non-enzymatic protein glycosylation is the addition of free carbonyls to the free amino groups of proteins, amino acids, lipoproteins and nucleic acids resulting in the formation of early glycation products. The early glycation products are also known as maillard reaction which undergoes dehydration, cyclization and rearrangement to form advanced glycation end-products (ages). By and large the researchers in the past have also established that glycation and the ages are responsible for most types of metabolic disorders, including diabetes mellitus, cancer, neurological disorders and aging. The amassing of ages in the tissues of neurodegenerative diseases shows its involvement in diseases. Therefore, it is likely that inhibition of glycation reaction may extend the lifespan of an individual. The hunt for inhibitors of glycation, mainly using in vitro models, has identified natural compounds able to prevent glycation, especially polyphenols and other natural antioxidants. Extrapolation of results of in vitro studies on the in vivo situation is not straightforward due to differences in the conditions and mechanism of glycation, and bioavailability problems. Nevertheless, existing data allow postulating that enrichment of diet in natural anti-glycating agents may attenuate glycation and, in consequence may halt the aging and neurological problems." This is exactly what happened to me and the degeneration of my brain due to the injury that i sustained years ago.

    I've lost 3 uncles and a brother-in-law to heart disease. My aunts and sister, all fed them the same food that I grew up on. The following is evidence of glycation's role in cardiovascular disease;

- **"ADVANCED GLYCATION END-PRODUCTS INDUCE APOPTOSIS OF VASCULAR SMOOTH MUSCLE CELLS: A MECHANISM FOR VASCULAR CALCIFICATION."**

    "Vascular calcification, especially medial artery calcification, is associated with cardiovascular death in patients with diabetes mellitus and chronic kidney disease (ckd). To determine the underlying mechanism of vascular calcification, we have demonstrated in our previous report that advanced glycation end-products (ages) stimulated calcium deposition in vascular smooth muscle cells (vsmcs) through excessive oxidative stress and phenotypic transition into osteoblastic cells. Since ages can induce apoptosis, in this study we investigated its role on vsmc apoptosis,

focusing mainly on the underlying mechanisms. A rat vsmc line (a7r5) was cultured and treated with glycolaldehyde-derived age-bovine serum albumin (age3-bsa). Apoptotic cells were identified by terminal deoxynucleotidyl transferased utp nick end labeling (tunel) staining. To quantify apoptosis, an enzyme-linked immunosorbent assay (elisa) for histone-complexed dna fragments was employed. Real-time pcr was performed to determine the mrna levels. Treatment of a7r5 cells with age3-bsa from 100 µg/ml concentration markedly increased apoptosis, which was suppressed by nox inhibitors. Age3-bsa significantly increased the mrna expression of nad (p)h oxidase components including nox4 and p22(phox), and these findings were confirmed by protein levels using immunofluorescence. Dihydroethidisum assay showed that compared with cbsa, age3-bsa increased reactive oxygen species level in a7r5 cells. Furthermore, age3-induced apoptosis was significantly inhibited by sirna-mediated knockdown of nox4 or p22 (phox). Double knockdown of nox4 and p22 (phox) showed a similar inhibitory effect on apoptosis as single gene silencing. Thus, our results demonstrated that nad (p)h oxidase-derived oxidative stress are involved in ages-induced apoptosis of vsmcs. These findings might be important to understand the pathogenesis of vascular calcification in diabetes and ckd."

Evidence of glycation in mental disorders like schizophrenia;

- ***"THE REGULATION OF SOLUBLE RECEPTOR FOR AGES CONTRIBUTES TO CARBOnYL STRESS IN SCHIZOPHRENIA."***
"Our previous study showed that enhanced carbonyl stress is closely related to schizophrenia. The endogenous secretory receptor for advanced glycation end-products (esrage) is a splice variant of the ager gene and is one of the soluble forms of rage. Esrage is considered to be a key molecule for alleviating the burden of carbonyl stress by entrapping advanced glycation end-products (ages). In the current study, we conducted genetic association analyses focusing on ager, in which we compared 212 schizophrenic patients to 214 control subjects. We also compared esrage levels among a subgroup of 104 patients and 89 controls and further carried out measurements of total circulating soluble rage (srage) in 25 patients and 49 healthy subjects. Although the genetic association study yielded inconclusive results, multiple regression analysis indicated that a specific haplotype composed of rs17846798, rs2071288, and a 63 bp deletion, which were in perfect linkage disequilibrium ($r^2 = 1$), and rs2070600 (gly82ser) were significantly associated with a marked decrease in serum esrage levels. Furthermore, compared to healthy subjects, schizophrenia showed significantly lower esrage ($p = 0.007$) and srage ($p = 0.03$)

levels, respectively. This is the first study to show that serum esrage levels are regulated by a newly identified specific haplotype in ager and that a subpopulation of schizophrenic patients are more vulnerable to carbonyl stress. Copyright © 2016 the authors. Published by elsevier inc. All rights reserved."

Have any of your doctors, psychiatrists, psychologists or therapists shared any of this information about protecting your mental or behavioral health, with you? None of mine did. They all preferred to prescribe medicines that would require more meds to counteract the effects of the side effects..

Evidence of glycation in renal disease and kidney cancer;

- **"GROWTH ARREST-SPECIFIC 2-LIKE PROTEIN 1 EXPRESSION IS UPREGULATED IN PODOCYTES THROUGH ADVANCED GLYCATION END-PRODUCTS."**

"BACKGROUND:
Growth arrest-specific 2-like protein 1 (gas2l1) protein is a member of the gas2 family of proteins, known to regulate apoptosis and cellular cytoskeleton reorganization in different cells. Recently we identified that gas2l1 gene expression in podocytes is influenced by advanced glycation end product-bovine serum albumin(age-bsa).
METHODS:
The study was performed employing cultured podocytes and diabetic (db/db) mice, a model of type 2 diabetes. Akbuminuria as well as urinary neutrophil gelatinase-associated lipocalin (ngal) excretion as measured with specific elisas. Gene expression was analyzed via semiquantitative and real-time polymerase chain reaction. The protein levels were determined by western blotting and immunostaining.
RESULTS:
We found that the gas2l1α isoform is expressed in podocytes. Treatment with age-bsa induced gas2l1α and gas2 mrna levels compared with controls incubated with non-glycated control bsa (co-bsa). Moreover, application of the recombinant soluble receptor of ages (srage), a competitor of cellular rage, reversed the age-bsa effect. Interestingly, age-bsa also increased the protein levels of gas2l1α in a rage-dependent manner but did not affect the gas2 expression. Periodic acid-schiff staining and albuminuria, as well as urinary ngal excretion, revealed that db/db mice progressively developed diabetic nephropathy with a renal accumulation of n_ε-carboxy-methyl-lysine (immunohistochemistry, western blots). Analyses of gas2l1α and gas2 proteins in diabetic mice revealed that both were significantly elevated relative to their non-diabetic

littermates. In addition, gas2l1α and gas2 proteins positively correlated with the accumulation of ages in the blood plasma of diabetic mice and the administration of srage in diabetic mice reduced the glomerular expression of both proteins.
CONCLUSIONS:
We show for the first time that the protein expression of gas2l1α in vitro and in vivo is regulated by the age-rage axis. The suppression of age ligation with their rage in diabetic mice with progressive nephropathy reversed the gas2l1α expression, thus suggesting a role of gas2l1α in the development of diabetic disease, which needs to be further elucidated. © the author 2016. Published by oxford university press on behalf of era-edta. All rights reserved"

Evidence of glycations influence in pancreatic cancer;

"ADVANCED GLYCATION END PRODUCTS IMPAIR GLUCOSE-STIMULATED INSULIN SECRETION OF A PANCREATIC B-CELL LINE INS-1-3 BY DISBURBANCE OF MICROTUBULE CYTOSKELETON VIA P38/MAPK ACTIVATION.

Advanced glycation end products (ages) are believed to be involved in diverse complications of diabetes mellitus. Overexposure to ages of pancreatic β-cells leads to decreased insulin secretion and cell apoptosis. Here, to understand the cytotoxicity of ages to pancreatic β-cells, we used ins-1-3 cells as a β-cell model to address this question, which was a subclone of ins-1 cells and exhibited a high level of insulin expression and high sensitivity to glucose stimulation. Exposed to large dose of ages, even though more insulin was synthesized, its secretion was significantly reduced from ins-1-3 cells. Further, ages treatment led to a time-dependent increase of depolymerized microtubules, which was accompanied by an increase of activated p38/mapk in ins-1-3 cells. Pharmacological inhibition of p38/mapk by sb202190 reversed microtubule depolymerization to a stabilized polymerization status but could not rescue the reduction of insulin release caused by ages. Taken together, these results suggest a novel role of ages-induced impairment of insulin secretion, which is partially due to a disturbance of microtubule dynamics that resulted from an activation of the p38/mapk pathway."

Amyloid plaque is at the root of most modern diseases, ranging from cancer to heart disease to arthritis to Alzheimer's disease;

- **"GLYCATION INDUCED GENERATION OF AMYLOID FIBRIL STRUCTURES BY GLUCOSE METABOLITES."**

"The non-enzymatic reaction (glycation) of reducing sugars with proteins has received increased interest in dietary and therapeutic research lately. In the present work, the impact of glycation on structural alterations of camel serum albumin (csa) by different glucose metabolites was studied. Glycation of csa was evaluated by specific fluorescence of advanced glycation end-products (ages) and determination of available amino groups. Further, conformational changes in csa during glycation were also studied using 8-analino 1-nephthlene sulfonic acid (ans) binding assay, circular dichroism (cd) and thermal analysis. Intrinsic fluorescence measurement of csa showed a 22 nm red shift after methylglyoxal treatment, suggesting glycation induced denaturation of csa. Rayleigh scattering analysis showed glycation induced turbidity and aggregation in csa. Furthermore, ans binding to native and glycated-csa reflected perturbation in the environment of hydrophobic residues. However, cd spectra did not reveal any significant modifications in the secondary structure of the glycated-csa. Thioflavin t (tht) fluorescence of csa increased after glycation, illustrated cross β-structure and amyloid formation. Transmission electron microscopy (tem) analysis further reaffirms the formation of aggregate and amyloid. In summary, glucose metabolites induced conformational changes in csa and produced aggregate and amyloid structures."

Is this the cure for Alzheimer's disease? No drugs needed for this one. This report is your evidence of glycations' involvement in Alzheimer's disease. If you remove the glycation, Alzheimer's can't happen; I don't know about you, but this speaks volumes, to me.

- **"HMGB1 AND THROMBIN MEDIATE THE BLOOD-BRAIN BARRIER DYSFUNCTION ACTING AS BIOMARKERS OF NEUROINFLAMMATION AND PROGRESSION TO NEURODEGENERATION IN ALZHEIMER'S DISEASE."**
BACKGROUND:
The blood-brain barrier (bbb) dysfunction represents an early feature of alzheimer's disease (ad) that precedes the hallmarks of amyloid beta (amyloid β) plaque deposition and neuronal neurofibrillary tangle (nft) formation. A damaged bbb correlates directly with neuroinflammation involving microglial activation and reactive astrogliosis, which is associated with increased expression and/or release of high-mobility group box protein 1 (hmgb1) and thrombin. However, the link between the presence of these molecules, bbb damage, and progression to neurodegeneration in ad is still elusive. Therefore, we aimed to profile and validate non-invasive clinical biomarkers of bbb dysfunction and

neuroinflammation to assess the progression to neurodegeneration in mild cognitive impairment (mci) and ad patients.
METHODS:
We determined the serum levels of various proinflammatory damage-associated molecules in aged control subjects and patients with mci or ad using validated elisa kits. We then assessed the specific and direct effects of such molecules on bbb integrity in vitro using human primary brain microvascular endothelial cells or a cell line.
RESULTS:
We observed a significant increase in serum hmgb1 and soluble receptor for advanced glycation end products (srage) that correlated well with amyloid beta levels in ad patients (vs. Control subjects). Interestingly, serum hmgb1 levels were significantly elevated in mci patients compared to controls or ad patients. In addition, as a marker of bbb damage, soluble thrombomodulin (stm) antigen, and activity were significantly (and distinctly) increased in mci and ad patients. Direct in vitro bbb integrity assessment further revealed a significant and concentration-dependent increase in paracellular permeability to dextrans by hmgb1 or α-thrombin, possibly through disruption of zona occludins-1 bands. Pre-treatment with anti-hmgb1 monoclonal antibody blocked hmgb1 effects and leaving bbb integrity intact.
CONCLUSIONS:
Our current studies indicate that thrombin and hmgb1 are causal proximate proinflammatory mediators of bbb dysfunction, while stm levels may indicate bbb endothelial damage; hmgb1 and srage might serve as clinical biomarkers for progression and/or therapeutic efficacy along the ad spectrum."

More evidence of the damaging effects of glycation;

- **_"THE FALSE ALARM HYPOTHESIS: FOOD ALLERGY IS ASSOCIATED WITH HIGH DIETARY ADVANCED GLYCATION END-PRODUCTS AND PROGLYCATING DIETARY SUGARS THAT MIMIC ALARMINS."_**
  "The incidence of food allergy has increased dramatically in the last few decades in westernized developed countries. We propose that the western lifestyle and diet promote innate danger signals and immune responses through production of "alarmins." alarmins are endogenous molecules secreted from cells undergoing nonprogrammed cell death that signal tissue and cell damage. High molecular group s (hmgb1) is a major alarmin that binds to the receptor for advanced glycation end-products (rage).
  Advanced glycation end-products (ages) are also present in foods.

We propose the "false alarm" hypothesis, in which ages that are present in or formed from the food in our diet are predisposing to food allergy. The western diet is high in ages, which are derived from cooked meat, oils, and cheese. Ages are also formed in the presence of a high concentration of sugars. We propose that a diet high in ages and age-forming sugars results in misinterpretation of a threat from dietary allergens, promoting the development of food allergy. Ages and other alarmins inadvertently prime innate signaling through multiple mechanisms, resulting in the development of allergic phenotypes. Current hypotheses and models of food allergy do not adequately explain the dramatic increase in food allergy in western countries. Dietary ages and age-forming sugars might be the missing link, a hypothesis supported by a number of convincing epidemiologic and experimental observations, as discussed in this article."

Evidence of the influence of glycation in dementia;

- **"INFLAMMATORY BIOMARKERS PREDICT DOMAIN-SPECIFIC COGNITIVE DECLINE IN OLDER ADULTS."**

"BACKGROUND:
Vascular risk factors, including inflammation, may contribute to dementia development. We investigated the associations between peripheral inflammatory biomarkers and cognitive decline in five domains (memory, construction, language, psychomotor speed, and executive function).
METHODS:
Community-dwelling older adults from the ginkgo evaluation of momory study (n = 1,159, aged 75 or older) free of dementia at baseline were included and followed for up to 7 years. Ten biomarkers were measured at baseline representing different sources of inflammation: vascular inflammation (pentraxin 3 and serum amyloid p), endothelial function (endothelin-1), metabolic function (adiponectin, resistin, and plasminogen activating inhibitor-1), oxidative stress (receptor for advanced glycation end products), and general inflammation (interleukin-6, interleukin-2, and interleukin-10). A combined z-score was created from these biomarkers to represent total inflammation across these sources. We utilized generalized estimating equations that included an interaction term between z-scores and time to assess the effect of inflammation on cognitive decline, adjusting for demographics (such as age, race/ethnicity, and sex), cardiovascular risk factors, and apolipoprotein e ε4 carrier status. A bonferroni-adjusted significance level of .01 was used. We explored associations between individual biomarkers and cognitive decline without adjustment for multiplicity.

RESULTS:
The combined inflammation z-score was significantly associated with memory and psychomotor speed (p < .01). Pentraxin 3, serum amyloid p, endothelin-1, and interleukin-2 were associated with change in at least one cognitive domain (p < .05).
CONCLUSION:
Our results suggest that total inflammation is associated with memory and psychomotor speed. In particular, systemic inflammation, vascular inflammation, and altered endothelial function may play roles in domain-specific cognitive decline of nondemented individuals.
*© the author 2016. Published by oxford university press on behalf of the gerontological society of america. All rights reserved. For permissions, please e-mail **journals.permissions@oup.com**.*

If you think that what you eat, can't have an effect on lung cancer your evidence of glycation in lung cancer;

- **"ADVANCEDGLYCATIONEND-PRODUCTS ENHANCE LUNG CANCER CELL INVASION AND MIGRATION."**
"Effects of carboxymethyllysine (cml) and pentosidine, two advanced glycation end-products (ages), upon invasion and migration in a549 and calu-6 cells, two non-small cell lung cancer (nsclc) cell lines were examined. Cml or pentosidine at 1, 2, 4, 8 or 16 µmol/l were added into cells. Proliferation, invasion, and migration were measured. Cml or pentosidine at 4-16 µmol/l promoted invasion and migration in both cell lines, and increased the production of reactive oxygen species, tumor necrosis factor-α, interleukin-6 and transforming growth factor-β1. Cml or pentosidine at 2-16 µmol/l up-regulated the protein expression of age receptor, p47(phox), intercellular adhesion molecule-1 and fibronectin in test nsclc cells. Matrix metalloproteinase-2 protein expression in a549 and calu-6 cells was increased by cml or pentosidine at 4-16 µmol/l. These two ages at 2-16 µmol/l enhanced nuclear factor κ-b (nf-κ b) p65 protein expression and p38 phosphorylation in a549 cells. However, cml or pentosidine at 4-16 µmol/l up-regulated nf-κb p65 and p-p38 protein expression in calu-6 cells. These findings suggest that cml and pentosidine, by promoting the invasion, migration, and production of associated factors, benefit nsclc metastasis."

This is the evidence of your back problems being caused by glycation. This study shows how the inflammatory responses to glycation causing vertebral disk degeneration. This is something, I get to deal with;

- **"IL-1B/HMGB1 SIGNALING PROMOTES THE INFLAMMATORY CYTOKINES RELEASE VIA TLR SIGNALING IN HUMAN INTERVERTEBRAL DISC CELLS."**

    "Inflammation and cytokines have been recognized to correlate with intervertebral disc (ivd) degeneration (idd), via mediating the development of clinical signs and symptoms. However, the regulation mechanism remains unclear. We aimed at investigating the regulatory role of interleukin (il)β and high mobility group box 1 (hmgb1) in the inflammatory response in human ivd cells and then explored the signaling pathways mediating such regulatory effect. Firstly, the promotion to inflammatory cytokines in ivd cells was examined with elisa method. And then western blot and real-time quantitative pcr were performed to analyze the expression of toll-like receptors (tlrs), receptors for advanced glycation endproducts (rage) and nf-κb signaling markers in the il-1β- or (and) hmgb1-treated ivd cells. Results demonstrated that either il-1β or hmgb1 promoted the release of the inflammatory cytokines such as prostaglandin e2 (pge2), tnf-α, il-6 and il-8 in human ivd cells. And the expression of matrix metalloproteinases (mmps) such as mmp-1, -3 and -9 was also additively up-regulated by il-1β and hmgb1. We also found such additive promotion to the expression of tlr-2, tlr-4 and rage, and the nf-κb signaling in intervertebral disc cells. In summary, our study demonstrated that il-1β and hmgb1 additively promotes the release of inflammatory cytokines and the expression of mmps in human ivd cells. The tlrs and rage and the nf-κb signaling were also additively promoted by il-1β and hmgb1. Our study implied that the additive promotion by il-1β and hmgb1 to inflammatory cytokines and mmps might aggravate the progression of idd."

Even unborn babies are not immune to the effects if glycation;

- **"ACCUMULATION OF ADVANCED GLYCATION END PRODUCTS INVOLVED IN INFLAMMATION AND CONTRIBUTING TO SEVERE PREECLAMPSIA, IN MATERNAL BLOOD, UMBILICAL BLOOD, AND PLACENTAL TISSUES."**

    "OBJECTIVE:
    To investigate the expression of advanced glycation end products (ages) and the receptor for age (rages) in maternal blood, umbilical blood and placental tissues in women with severe preeclampsia (spe) as well as any association with inflammatory processes.
    METHODS:
    The expressions of ages, rage, tumor necrosis factor-alpha (tnf)-α and vascular cell adhesion molecule-1 (vcam)-1 in placental tissues were measured using immunohistochemistry. The levels of ages, rage, tnf-α, and vcam-1 in maternal blood, umbilical blood and

placental extracts were assessed using enzyme-linked immunosorbent assays. Placental rage, tnf-α, and vcam-1 mrna expression levels were determined by pcr. Placental ages, rage, tnf-α and vcam-1 protein levels were determined by western blotting.
RESULTS:
The levels of ages, tnf-α, and vcam-1 in the maternal tissues and umbilical blood were significantly higher in the spe group than in the normal pregnancy (np) controls (p < 0.05). The serum level of srage in the umbilical blood was lower in the spe group than in the np controls (p < 0.05), while srage was higher in the maternal blood of spe than in the np (p < 0.05). The maternal serum levels of ages were positively correlated with that of tnf-α and vcam-1 in the maternal blood. There were no correlations between the levels of rage, tnf-α or vcam-1 in maternal blood or umbilical serum. There were no correlations between the levels of srage and tnf-α or vcam-1 in maternal blood or umbilical serum. The levels of ages were positively correlated with those of tnf-α and vcam-1 in placental lysates.
CONCLUSION:
Ages and rage appear to act as important mediators in regulating the inflammatory pathways of preeclampsia."

Ovarian cancer is a consequence of glycation as evidenced in the next study;

- **S100B MEDIATES STEMNESS OF OVARIAN CANCER STEM-LIKE CELLS THROUGH INHIBITING P53.**
"S100b is one of the members of the s100 protein family and is involved in the progression of a variety of cancers. Ovarian cancer is driven by cancer stem-like cells (cslcs) that are involved in tumor genesis, metastasis, chemo-resistance, and relapse. We then hypothesized that s100b might exert pro-tumor effects by regulating ovarian cslcs stemness, a key characteristic of cslcs. First, we observed the high expression of s100b in ovarian cancer specimens when compared to that in normal ovary. The s100b upregulation associated with more advanced tumor stages, poorer differentiation and poorer survival. In addition, elevated s100b expression correlated with increased expression of stem cell markers including cd133, nanog and oct4. Then, we found that s100b was preferentially expressed in cd133⁺ ovarian cslcs derived from both ovarian cancer cell lines and primary tumors of patients. More importantly, we revealed that s100b knockdown suppressed the in vitro self-renewal and in vivo tumorigenicity of ovarian cslcs and decreased their expression of stem cell markers. S100b ectopic expression endowed non-cslcs with stemness, which has been

demonstrated with both in vitro and in vivo experiments. Mechanically, we demonstrated that the underlying mechanism of s100b-mediated effects on cslcs stemness was not dependent on its binding with a receptor for advanced glycation end products (rage), but might be through intracellular regulation, through the inhibition of p53 expression and phosphorylation. In conclusion, our results elucidate the importance of s100b in the maintenance of ovarian cslcs stemness, which might provide a promising therapeutic target for ovarian cancer. Stem cells 2016."

This study looks at the AGEs responsible for inflammatory bowel disease and Rheumatoid arthritis;

- **"S100A8/A9: FROM BASIC SCIENCE TO CLINICAL APPLICATION."**
"Neutrophils and monocytes belong to the first line of immune defense cells and are recruited to sites of inflammation during infection or sterile injury. Both cells contain huge amounts of the heterodimeric protein s100a8/a9 in their cytoplasm. S100a8/a9 belongs to the ca^{2+} binding s100 protein family and has recently gained a lot of interest as a critical alarmin modulating the inflammatory response after its release (extracellular s100a8/a9) from neutrophils and monocytes. Extracellular s100a8/a9 interacts with the pattern recognition receptors toll-like receptor 4 (tlr4) and receptor for advanced **glycation** endproducts (rage) promoting cell activation and recruitment. Besides its biological function, s100a8/a9 (also known as myeloid-related protein 8/14, mrp8/14) was identified as an interesting biomarker to monitor disease activity in chronic inflammatory disorders including inflammatory bowel disease and rheumatoid arthritis. Furthermore, s100a8/a9 has been tested successfully in pre-clinical imaging studies to localize sites of infection or sterile injury. Finally, recent evidence using small molecule inhibitors for s100a8/a9 also suggests that blocking s100a8/a9 activity exerts beneficial effects on disease activity in animal models of autoimmune diseases including multiple sclerosis, systemic lupus erythematosus, rheumatoid arthritis and inflammatory bowel disease. This review will provide a comprehensive and detailed overview into the structure and biological function of s100a8/a9 and also will give an outlook in terms of diagnostic and therapeutic applications targeting s100a8/a9".

Remember, when I said that inflammation couldn't exist without glycation? Here's your evidence;

- **"THE EMERGING ROLE OF HMGB1 IN NEUROPATHIC PAIN: A POTENTIAL THERAPEUTIC TARGET FOR NEUROINFLAMMATION."**
"Neuropathic pain (npp) is an intolerable, persistent, and specific type of long-term pain. It is considered to be a direct consequence of pathological changes affecting the somatosensory system and can be debilitating for affected patients. Despite recent progress and growing interest in understanding the pathogenesis of the disease, npp still presents a major diagnostic and therapeutic challenge. High mobility group box 1 (hmgb1) mediates inflammatory and immune reactions in nervous system and emerging evidence reveals that hmgb1 plays an essential role in neuroinflammation through receptors such as toll-like receptors (tlr), receptor for advanced **glycation** end products (rage), c-x-x motif chemokines receptor 4 (cxcr4), and n-methyl-d-aspartate (nmda) receptor. In this review, we present evidence from studies that address the role of hmgb1 in npp. First, we review studies aimed at determining the role of hmgb1 in npp and discuss the possible mechanisms underlying hmgb1-mediated npp progression where receptors for hmgb1 are involved. Then we review studies that address hmgb1 as a potential therapeutic target for npp."

Perhaps the most damning report was issued in January of 1984, yet nothing was mentioned about this report; it was one of the first indications of what glycation does to the body and with a major cause of glycation being glucose or sugar, I have to wonder why the FDA didn't say anything about it. Why weren't we, at least, informed about this study?

- **"COLLAGEN AGING IN VITRO BY NONENZYMATIC GLYCOSYLATION AND BROWNING."**
Aging and diabetes mellitus are associated with cross-linking and nonenzymatic glycosylation of collagen. Incubation of tendon fibers with reducing sugars results in increased breaking time in urea similar to that seen in aging, and in nonenzymatic glycosylation and browning. Effect of a sugar is proportional to the amount of sugar available in the open chain form. The increase in breaking time correlates with the appearance of chromophores characteristic of cross linked browning products. Collagen altered by nonenzymatic browning may play a role in some age-like major complications of diabetes."

This evidence of glycation's role in atherosclerosis was in this study submitted in May 1988. What has your doctor told you about this study?

- **"DIMINISHED ADHESION OF ENDOTHELIAL AORTIC CELLS ON FIBRONECTIN AND COLLAGEN LAYERS AFTER NONENZYMATIC GLYCATION."**
  Adhesion of bovine endothelial cells on fibronectin and collagen before and after nonenzymatic glycation in vitro has been studied. Nonenzymatic glycation of these proteins reduced their ability to bind endothelial cells. Furthermore, nonenzymatically glycated fibronectin failed to bind to normal and nonenzymatically glycated gelatin and to fibrin. So gelatin and fibrin sepharoses can be used to separate highly glycated fibronectins from fibronectins with a low degree of nonenzymatic glucose substitution. Sodium dodecylsulfate polyacrylamide gel electrophoresis did not demonstrate a covalent cross-link between nonenzymatically glycated fibronectins. These results present further evidence for the role of nonenzymatic glycation of proteins in the development of vascular complications in long-term diabetes and of atherosclerosis.

This shows the damage done by glycation on the blood. I posted this study because I wanted to note the date of this study is July 29, 1988, forty years ago, Yet have you heard anything about this?

- **"GLYCATED HEMOGLOBINS"**
  "The association between elevated levels of glycated hemoglobins and diabetes mellitus has been known for twenty years. Since then the determination of glycated hemoglobins has become a valuable tool for the objective assessment of long-term glycemia in diabetic patients. The marked clinical interest in reliable measurements of glycated hemoglobins has stimulated the development and perfection of the necessary methodology. Limitations of the techniques have led to an investigation of the underlying causes. Some of them led to the recognition of processes that were not known to occur in vivo before, such as glycation at sites other than the amino terminus of the beta-chains, modification of hemoglobin by reactants other than glucose or the existence of labile hemoglobin adducts. With ideal methodology, these features would have gone unnoticed. Furthermore, the determination of glycated hemoglobin in large populations of diabetic patients has to lead to the discovery of new, clinically silent mutant hemoglobins. Today, the routine determination of glycated hemoglobins in diabetic patients probably represents the broadest screening for mutant hemoglobins. The experience with glycated hemoglobins shows that overcoming difficulties in their determination, and progress in biomedical research, are closely intertwined.

This study shows how proteins exposed to glucose undergoes oxidative stress, the basis of aging;

- **"AUTOXIDATIVE GLYCOSYLATION "FREE RADICALS AND GLYCATION THEORY."**
  "Studies have shown that glycation in vitro is complicated by the ability of glucose to oxidize, in the presence of trace amounts of a transition metal, generating protein-reactive ketoaldehydes, hydrogen peroxide, and diverse free radicals. Protein exposed to glucose undergoes fragmentational and conformational alterations, and these, as well as thiol oxidation, appear to be caused by hydroxyl radicals. Glycofluorophore formation is dependent upon ketoaldehyde formation. It is suggested that glucose autoxidation contributes to oxidative stress in pathophysiology associated with diabetes and ageing via this newly described process of "autoxidative glycosylation".

The following report from Oct 30, 1981, shows the effects of glycation on cholesterol, LDL particles particularly and how it leads to atherosclerosis ;

- **"NONENZYMATIC GLYCOSYLATION OF LOW-DENSITY LIPOPROTEINS IN VITRO. EFFECTS ON CELL-INTERACTIVE PROPERTIES."**
  Atherosclerosis occurs at an accelerated rate in patients with diabetes mellitus. Since some proteins undergo nonenzymatic glycosylation in diabetic patients and because certain chemical modifications of low-density lipoproteins produced alterations in their interactions with certain cultured cells, a fact that may be relevant to atherogenesis, we investigated the effect of in vitro glycosylation on cell-related properties of low-density lipoproteins. Glycosylation was carried out by incubating ldl (1-10 mg ldl-protein/ml) with glucose (0-100 mm) in 0.5 m phosphate buffer, ph 8.0, at 37 degrees c. The amount of glucose incorporated into ldl after 1-2 wk of incubation was estimated to be in the range of 1-10 mol/mol ldl-protein. Amino acid analysis of glycosylated ldl showed that glucose was covalently bound to lysine residues. In studies with cultured human fibroblasts, glycosylated ldl was internalized and degraded significantly less than control ldl, in proportion to the estimated degree of glycosylation (12% of control for the most extensively glycosylated ldl). Glycosylation of ldl also impaired significantly its ability to stimulate cholesteryl ester synthesis by cultured fibroblasts. Glycosylated ldl did not stimulate cholesteryl ester synthesis in rat peritoneal macrophages. If glycosylation of ldl occurs in diabetic

patients, some pathophysiologic consequences related to the increased incidence of atherosclerosis in these patients may result.

In 1981 this was discovered, yet it's been 35 years since then and yet few people are aware of this. My question is, why? Maybe I should ask the sugar industry.

The following study shows how the adhesive qualities of glucose create fibrinogen, which becomes a target for glycation;

- **"POLYMERISATION AND CROSSLINKING OF FIBRIN MONOMERS IN DIABETES MELLITUS."**
Polymerisation and crosslinking of fibrin monomers were studied in 35 healthy volunteers and in 42 poorly controlled diabetic patients. Polymerisation did not show any difference between control subjects (n = 10) and diabetic patients (n = 11) (p greater than 0.1), although fibrinogen was 35% more glycated in the diabetic patients (p less than 0.001). Alpha chain crosslinking in the diabetic patients, however, was impaired as is shown from an increase in intermediate alpha polymers with a concomitant decrease in alpha monomer disappearance. A significant positive correlation was found between the degree of glycation of fibrinogen and the defective alpha chain polymerization (r = 0.86, p less than 0.005). These results were consistent with the results of thrombin and reptilase experiments. The reaction rate with reptilase did not show any difference between the two groups (p greater than 0.1), whereas the reaction rate with thrombin was significantly slower in the diabetic group compared to the control subjects (p less than 0.001). Purified fibrin clots obtained from the diabetic patients were more susceptible to plasmin than clots obtained from control subjects. It is concluded that in poorly controlled diabetic patients polymerization of fibrin monomers is normal, but crosslinking of the alpha chains is impaired, leading to a higher susceptibility of the clots to plasmin degradation.

From Wikipedia on Fibrinogen;

fibrinogen (factor i) is a **glycoprotein** *in* **vertebrates** *that helps in the formation of blood clots. it consists of a linear array of three nodules held together by a very thin thread which is estimated to have a diameter between 8 and 15* **angstrom** *(å). the two end nodules are alike but the center one is slightly smaller. measurements of shadow lengths indicate that nodule diameters are in the range 50 to 70 å. the length of the dried molecule is 475 ± 25 å.*

With apoB being at the root of almost all modern disease, the following report is of vital importance;

- **"EFFECT OF LOW-DENSITY LIPOPROTEIN ON THE IMMUNOLOGICAL DETERMINATION GLYCATION OF APOLIPOPROTEIN B."**
"Non-enzymatic glycation of low-density lipoprotein (ldl) may contribute to the premature atherogenesis of patients with diabetes mellitus. To assess whether glycation of apolipoprotein b, the predominant protein of ldl, interferes with the ability to immunologically quantify this protein, we prepared and purified glycated ldl by incubating normal plasma samples with high concentrations of glucose. Although both the plasma and the ldl specimens incubated with glucose contained significantly more glycated protein than control specimens, the quantitative interaction of an apolipoprotein b-specific antibody with glycated vs nonglycated ldl was not significantly different. We conclude that apolipoprotein b can be accurately quantified immunologically despite the presence of clinically excessive degrees of ldl glycation."

I included the following study from November 1989 because of its explanation of how glycation is responsible for inflammation;

- **'CHANGES IN CONCANAVALIN A-REACTIVE PROTEINS IN INFLAMMATORY DISORDERS."**
"Quantitative changes of concanavalin a (con a)-reactive proteins in serum samples obtained from rats with induced inflammation and from patients with inflammatory and autoimmune diseases were examined by use of lectin blots. Treatment of rats with a single dose of fermented yeast to induce inflammation caused an extensive increase in con a-reactivity. These changes were time-dependent and were similar in both sexes of the animals. When we examined serum samples obtained from patients with various inflammatory disorders for their con a-reactive proteins as compared with normal donors, we noted that the con a-reactivity increased in patients with rheumatoid arthritis and systemic lupus erythematosus. Among all the glycoproteins examined by lectin blots with use of con a, a set of five proteins was selected for detailed analysis by densitometric scanning. These included alpha 2-macroglobulin, p-150, p-95, p-40, and p-35, of mr 180,000, 150,000, 95,000, 40,000, and 35,000, respectively, by sodium dodecyl sulfate-polyacrylamide gel electrophoresis under reducing conditions. Densitometric scanning analysis of the lectin blots revealed that the con a-reactivity of these proteins increased during inflammation. Because alpha 2-

macroglobulin is not an acute-phase protein in humans, an increase in con a staining of this protein suggested that altered glycation is associated with autoimmune diseases. Thus, the study of changes in con a-reactive proteins in human sera may facilitate our understanding of the etiology and pathophysiology of autoimmune diseases."

- **"CLINICAL VALUE OF HIGH MOBILITY GROUP BOX 1 AND THE RECEPTOR FOR ADVANCED GLYCATION END-PRODUCTS IN HEAD AND NECK CANCER: A SYSTEMATIC REVIEW."**
"ABSTRACT
Introduction   high mobility group box 1 is a versatile protein involved in gene transcription, extracellular signaling, and response to inflammation. Extracellularly, high mobility group box 1 binds to several receptors, notably the receptor **for** advanced glycation end-products. Expression of high mobility group box 1 and the receptor for advanced glycation end-products has been described in many cancers. Objectives   to systematically review the available literature using pubmed and web of science to evaluate the clinical value of high mobility group box 1 and the receptor for advanced glycation end-products in head and neck squamous cell carcinomas. Data synthesis   a total of eleven studies were included in this review. High mobility group box 1 overexpression is associated with poor prognosis and many clinical and pathological characteristics of head and neck squamous cell carcinomas patients. Additionally, the receptor for advanced glycation end-products demonstrates potential value as a clinical indicator of tumor angiogenesis and advanced staging. In diagnosis, high mobility group box 1 demonstrates low sensitivity. Conclusion   high mobility group box 1 and the receptor for advanced glycation end-products are associated with clinical and pathological characteristics of head and neck squamous cell carcinomas. Further investigation of the prognostic and diagnostic value of these molecules is warranted."

- **"GLYCOSYLATED LIPOPROTEIN. "**
"Diabetes is frequently associated with cardiovascular diseases (coronary heart disease, cerebrovascular disease, peripheral vascular disease), and several risk factors have been proposed. Recent studies have strengthened the importance of chronic hyperglycemia because this modifies a variety of circulating substances including lipoproteins, and the glycosylated ones can be involved in the process of accelerating atherosclerosis. In this review, previous studies indicating the significance of glycosylated lipoproteins in the progression of atherosclerosis were overviewed. We also discussed age (advanced glycation end

products) which may play an important role of atherogenesis in diabetes.

The most recent study, submitted in october 2016 reveals some of the known damage that glycation is responsible for;

- **"RELATIONSHIP BETWEEN PLASMA GLYCATION WITH MEMBRANE MODIFICATION, OXIDATIVE STRESS AND EXPRESSION OF GLUCOSE TRASPORTER-1 IN TYPE 2 DIABETES PATIENTS WITH VASCULAR COMPLICATIONS."**

BACKGROUND OF STUDY:
Enhanced protein glycation in diabetes causes irreversible cellular damage through membrane modifications. Erythrocytes are persistently exposed to plasma glycated proteins; however, little is known about its consequences on the membrane. The aim of this study was to examine the relationship between plasma protein glycation with erythrocyte membrane modifications in type 2 diabetes patients with and without vascular complications.
METHOD:
We recruited 60 healthy controls, 85 type 2 diabetic mellitus (dm) and 75 type 2 diabetic patients with complications (dmc). Levels of plasma glycation adduct with antioxidants (fructosamine, protein carbonyl, β-amyloids, thiol groups, total antioxidant status), erythrocyte membrane modifications (protein carbonyls, β-amyloids, free amino groups, erythrocyte fragility), antioxidant profile (gsh, catalase, lipid peroxidation) and glut-1 expression were quantified.
RESULT:
Compared with controls, dm and dmc patients had a significantly higher level of glycation adducts, erythrocyte fragility, lipid peroxidation and glut-1 expression whereas declined levels of plasma and cellular antioxidants. Correlation studies revealed the positive association of membrane modifications with erythrocyte sedimentation rate, fragility, peroxidation whereas the negative association with free amino groups, glutathione, and catalase.
CONCLUSION:
Our data suggest that plasma glycation is associated with oxidative stress, glut-1 expression and erythrocyte fragility in dm patients. This may further contribute to the progression of vascular complications.

Has anybody ever shared how cataracts manifest themselves in your eyes? Evidence of the glycative effects in Cataracts are in the following report;

- **"NONENZYMATIC GLYCATION OF HUMAN LENS CRYSTALLIN. EFFECT OF AGING AND DIABETES MELLITUS "**
- *Garlick RL, Mazer JS, Chylack LT Jr, Tung WH, Bunn HF.*

  We have examined the nonenzymatic glycation of human lens crystallin, an extremely long-lived protein, from 16 normal human ocular lenses 0.2-99 yr of age, and from 11 diabetic lenses 52-82-yr-old. The glucitol-lysine (glc-lys) content of soluble and insoluble crystallin was determined after reduction with h-borohydride followed by acid hydrolysis, boronic acid affinity chromatography, and high-pressure cation exchange chromatography. Normal lens crystallin, soluble and insoluble, had 0.028 +/- 0.011 nanomoles glc-lys per nanomole crystallin monomer. Soluble and insoluble crystallins had equivalent levels of glycation. The content of glc-lys in normal lens crystallin increased with age in a linear fashion. Thus, the nonenzymatic glycation of nondiabetic lens crystallin may be regarded as a biological clock. The diabetic lens crystallin samples (n = 11) had a higher content of glc-lys (0.070 +/- 0.034 nmol/nmol monomer). Over an age range comparable to that of the control samples, the diabetic crystallin samples contained about twice as much glc-lys. The glc-lys content of the diabetic lens crystallin samples did not increase with lens age.

This last study looked at the effects of glycation on your eyes and the cataracts, it's responsible for. Yes, glycation and a glucose diet will buy you cataracts. My mother had two of them. A good friend who loved to eat her bread had cataracts in both of her eyes as well. What's interesting, this person was always complaining of headaches and stomachaches, both manifestations of an ecc diet. Again, here is more evidence of the glycative and addictive effects of a grain diet. *The following report provides evidence of glycation's role in leukemia.*

- ***EXTRACELLULAR HMGB1 PROMOTES DIFFERENTIATION OF NURSE-LIKE CELLS IN CHRONIC LYMPHOCYTIC LEUKEMIA.***

  "Chronic lymphocytic leukemia (cll) is a disease of an accumulation of mature b cells that are highly dependent on the microenvironment for maintenance and expansion. However, little is known regarding the mechanisms whereby cll cells create their favorable microenvironment for survival. High-mobility group protein b-1 (hmgb1) is a highly conserved nuclear protein that can be actively secreted by innate immune cells and passively released by injured or dying cells. We found significantly increased hmgb1 levels in the plasma of cll patients compared with healthy controls, and hmgb1 concentration is associated with absolute lymphocyte count. We, therefore, sought to determine potential roles of hmgb1 in

modulating the cll microenvironment. Cll cells passively released hmgb1, and the timing and concentrations of hmgb1 in the medium were associated with differentiation of nurse-like cells (nlcs). Higher cd68 expression in cll lymph nodes, one of the markers for nlcs, was associated with shorter overall survival of cll patients. Hmgb1-mediated nlc differentiation involved internalization of both, receptor for advanced glycation end products (rage) and toll-like receptor-9 (tlr9). Differentiation of nlcs can be prevented by blocking the hmgb1-rage-tlr9 pathway. In conclusion, this study demonstrates for the first time that cll cells might modulate their microenvironment by releasing hmgb1."

After searching these last few disorders I got a yen to search any disorder & glycation, and glycation turned up in everything, even halitosis. The following report shows its involvement in stomach ulcers. I originally searched just ulcers and got back 30 studies showing involvement. The first few studies in the list were reports on foot ulcers, so I searched stomach ulcers and found 3 studies, the following report was the first;

- ***HIGH-MOBILITY GROUP BOX 1 INHIBITS GASTRIC ULCER HEALING THROUGH TOLL-LIKE RECEPTOR4 AND RECEPTOR FOR ADVANCED GLYCATION END PRODUCTS***
  "*High-mobility group box 1 (HMGB1) was initially discovered as a nuclear protein that interacts with DNA as a chromatin-associated non-histone protein to stabilize nucleosomes and to regulate the transcription of many genes in the nucleus. Once leaked or actively secreted into the extracellular environment, HMGB1 activates inflammatory pathways by stimulating multiple receptors, including Toll-like receptor (TLR) 2, TLR4, and receptor for advanced glycation end products (RAGE), leading to tissue injury. Although HMGB1's ability to induce inflammation has been well documented, no studies have examined the role of HMGB1 in wound healing in the gastrointestinal field. The aim of this study was to evaluate the role of HMGB1 and its receptors in the healing of gastric ulcers. We also investigated which receptor among TLR2, TLR4, or RAGE mediates HMGB1's effects on ulcer healing. Gastric ulcers were induced by serosal application of acetic acid in mice, and gastric tissues were processed for further evaluation. The induction of ulcer increased the immunohistochemical staining of cytoplasmic HMGB1 and elevated serum HMGB1 levels. Ulcer size, myeloperoxidase (MPO) activity, and the expression of tumor necrosis factor α (TNFα) mRNA peaked on day 4. Intraperitoneal administration of HMGB1 delayed ulcer healing and elevated MPO activity and TNFα expression. In contrast, administration of anti-*

HMGB1 antibody promoted ulcer healing and reduced MPO activity and TNFα expression. TLR4 and RAGE deficiency enhanced ulcer healing and reduced the level of TNFα, whereas ulcer healing in TLR2 knockout (KO) mice was similar to that in wild-type mice. In TLR4 KO and RAGE KO mice, exogenous HMGB1 did not affect ulcer healing and TNFα expression. Thus, we showed that HMGB1 is a complicating factor in the gastric ulcer healing process, which acts through TLR4 and RAGE to induce excessive inflammatory responses."

The following study from Aug 11, 2015, is proof that glycation starts in the mouth. As soon as you eat, the glucose in the food starts glycating your saliva, as saliva is a digestive juice and this is where digestion starts. Although I suspected this, this is the smoking gun article proving glycation's destructive effects. This showed up in prehistoric times as well, it's commonly known to archeologists when prehistoric man started eating a wheat-based diet, it shows up in their teeth in the form of cavities and missing teeth, that didn't show up in earlier man who didn't have a diet in grains.

- **BLOOD CONTAMINATION IN SALIVA: IMPACT ON THE MEASUREMENT OF SALIVARY OXIDATIVE STRESS MARKERS.**
"Salivary oxidative stress markers represent a promising tool for monitoring of oral diseases. Saliva can often be contaminated by blood, especially in patients with periodontitis. The aim of our study was to examine the impact of blood contamination on the measurement of salivary oxidative stress markers. Saliva samples were collected from 10 healthy volunteers and were artificially contaminated with blood (final concentration 0.001-10%).
Next, saliva was collected from 12 gingivitis and 10 control patients before and after dental hygiene treatment. Markers of oxidative stress were measured in all collected saliva samples. Advanced oxidation protein products (AOPP), advanced glycation end products (AGEs), and antioxidant status were changed in 1% blood-contaminated saliva. Salivary AOPP were increased in control and patients after dental treatment (by 45.7% and 34.1%, $p < 0.01$). Salivary AGEs were decreased in patients after microinjury (by 69.3%, $p < 0.001$). Salivary antioxidant status markers were decreased in both control and patients after dental treatment ($p < 0.05$ and $p < 0.01$). One % blood contamination biased concentrations of salivary oxidative stress markers. Saliva samples with 1% blood contamination are visibly discolored and can be excluded from analyses without any specific biochemic detection of blood constituents. Salivary markers of oxidative stress were significantly altered in blood-contaminated saliva in control and patients with gingivitis after dental hygiene treatment."

- **_PULMONARY RECEPTOR FOR ADVANCED GLYCATION END-PRODUCTS PROMOTES ASTHMA PATHOGENESIS THROUGH IL-33 AND ACCUMULATION OF GROUP 2 INNATE LYMPHOID CELLS._**

  Abstract

  BACKGROUND:

  Single nucleotide polymorphisms in the human gene for the receptor for advanced glycation end-products(RAGE) are associated with an increased incidence of asthma. RAGE is highly expressed in the lung and has been reported to play a vital role in the pathogenesis of murine models of asthma/allergic airway inflammation (AAI) by promoting expression of the type 2 cytokines IL-5 and IL-13. IL-5 and IL-13 are prominently secreted by group 2 innate lymphoid cells (ILC2s), which are stimulated by the proallergic cytokine IL-33.

  OBJECTIVE:

  We sought to test the hypothesis that pulmonary RAGE is necessary for allergen-induced ILC2 accumulation in the lung.

  METHODS:

  AAI was induced in wild-type and RAGE knockout mice by using IL-33, house dust mite extract, or Alternaria alternata extract. RAGE's lung-specific role in type 2 responses was explored with bone marrow chimeras and induction of gastrointestinal type 2 immune responses.

  RESULTS:

  RAGE was found to drive AAI by promoting IL-33 expression in response to allergen and by coordinating the inflammatory response downstream of IL-33. Absence of RAGE impedes pulmonary accumulation of ILC2s in models of AAI. Bone marrow chimera studies suggest that pulmonary parenchymal, but not hematopoietic, RAGE has a central role in promoting AAI. In contrast to the lung, the absence of RAGE does not affect IL-33-induced ILC2 influx in the spleen, type 2cytokine production in the peritoneum, or mucus hypersecretion in the gastrointestinal tract.

  CONCLUSIONS:

  For the first time, this study demonstrates that a parenchymal factor, RAGE, mediates lung-specific accumulation of ILC2s.

- **_CELIAC DISEASE AND IMMUNOLOGICAL DISORDERS._**

  Out of 314 patients with coeliac disease, 63 had associated disorders of known or suspected immunological cause (excluding aphthous stomatitis and dermatitis herpetiformis). Autoimmune diseases appeared to occur more often in patients with coeliac disease than in the normal population, 52 such diseases being found in 45 patients. Of individual disorders, diabetes mellitus, thyroid diseases, and ulcerative colitis seemed to be more common than expected. Atopy (asthma and eczema) occurred in 7% of the patients. Most of these immunological disorders developed when the patients were on normal diet. A gluten-free diet and virtually normal jejunum did not prevent their development, and the diet had a little ameliorating effect on their course apart from an occasional dramatic improvement in atopic patients.

The following report shows the effects of glycation in Fibromyalgia from May 2009. Do you suffer from fibromyalgia? Has your doctor shared this information with you? If not, why?:

- **_ABNORMAL PAIN MODULATION IN PATIENTS WITH SPATIALLY DISTRIBUTED CHRONIC PAIN: FIBROMYALGIA_**

  Many chronic pain syndromes including fibromyalgia, irritable bowel syndrome, chronic fatigue syndrome, migraine headache, chronic back pain, and complex regional pain syndrome are associated with hypersensitivity to painful stimuli and with reduced endogenous pain inhibition. These findings suggest that modulation of pain-related information may be related to the onset and/or maintenance of chronic pain. Although pain sensitivity and pain inhibition are normally distributed in the general population, they are not useful as reliable predictors of future pain. The combination of heightened pain sensitivity and reduced pain-inhibition, however, appears to predispose individuals to greater risk for increased acute clinical pain (e.g., postoperative pain). It is unknown at this time whether such pain processing abnormalities may also place individuals at increased risk for chronic pain. Psychophysical methods, including heat sensory and pressure pain testing, have become increasingly available and can be used for the evaluation of pain sensitivity and pain inhibition. However, long-term prospective studies in the general population are lacking which could yield insight into the role of heightened pain sensitivity and pain disinhibition for the development of chronic pain disorders like fibromyalgia.

The studies below show glycation's responsibility in Idiopathic pulmonary fibrosis (IPF) and non-specific interstitial pneumonia (NSIP). This study is from NIH's PMC is the second of 135 studies done on glycation and IPF. They were published on the 15th of Dec 2013 and Nov5 2016.

- **ADVANCED GLYCATION END-PRODUCTS AND RECEPTOR FOR ADVANCED GLYCATION END-PRODUCTS EXPRESSION IN PATIENTS WITH IDIOPATHIC PULMONARY FIBROSIS AND NSIP**

    "Advanced glycation end products (AGEs) are associated with the pathogenesis of various diseases. AGEs induce excess accumulation of extracellular matrix and expression of profibrotic cytokines. In addition, studies on the receptor for advanced glycation end products (RAGE) have shown that the ligand-RAGE interaction activates several intracellular signaling cascades associated with several fibrotic diseases. We investigated the expression of AGEs and RAGE in samples from patients with idiopathic pulmonary fibrosis (IPF) and non-specific interstitial pneumonia (NSIP). Lung tissues and plasma samples from patients with IPF (n=10), NSIP (n=10), and control subjects (n=10) were obtained. Expression of AGEs and RAGE was determined by immunofluorescence assay of lung tissue. Circulating AGEs were measured by Western blot and enzyme-linked immunosorbent assay. Lungs with IPF showed strong expression for both AGEs and RAGE compared to that in NSIP and controls. However, no difference in AGE or RAGE expression was observed in lungs with NSIP compared to that in the controls. Levels of circulating AGEs also increased significantly in lungs of patients with IPF compared to those with NSIP and normal control. The increased AGE-RAGE interaction may play an n important role in the pathogenesis of IPF.

    "None of the patients had diabetes. Patients with NSIP were younger than control subjects and those with IPF. Patients with IPF and NSIP had decreased pulmonary function compared to control subjects. Patients with IPF had high plasma AGE levels and a poor prognosis for survival. No correlation was observed between plasma AGE levels and clinical parameters, including survival (data not shown)".

- **AGE AND RAGE EXPRESSION IN LUNG TISSUES OF PATIENTS WITH NSIP AND IPF**

    IPF lungs strongly expressed both AGE and RAGE compared to NSIP and control lungs. However, no difference in AGE or RAGE expression was observed in NSIP compared to control lungs. We performed staining with macrophage-specific Iba1 and OX42 to localize AGE expression in IPF lungs and observed a merged state with AGE-modified albumin Immunofluorescence staining for both Iba1 and OX42 showed that macrophages contained AGE-modified albumin.

- **INCREASED AGE-RAGE RATIO IN IDIOPATHIC PULMONARY FIBROSIS**
"Our study demonstrates an increase of AGEs together with a decrease of RAGEs in IPF lungs, compared with control samples. Two specific AGEs involved in aging, pentosidine and Nε-Carboxymethyl lysine, were significantly increased in IPF samples. The immunohistochemistry identified higher staining of AGEs related to extracellular matrix (ECM) proteins and the apical surface of the alveolar epithelial cells (AECs) surrounding fibroblast foci in fibrotic lungs. On the other hand, RAGE location was present at the cell membrane of AECs in control lungs, while it was almost missing in pulmonary fibrotic tissue. In addition, in vitro cultures showed that the effect of AGEs on cell viability was different for AECs and fibrotic fibroblasts. AGEs decreased cell viability in AECs, even at low concentration, while fibroblast viability was less affected. Furthermore, fibroblast to myofibroblast transformation could be enhanced by ECM glycation."
"All of these findings suggest a possible role of the increased ratio AGEs-RAGEs in IPF, which could be a relevant accelerating aging tissue reaction in the abnormal wound healing of the lung fibrotic process."

IPF is still thought to have no known cause, yet I know if one thing were removed from the equation, it wouldn't exist. What is that one thing? You guessed it, glucose, the primary cause of glycation. What would happen if you removed glycation from this equation? Are you asking yourself, can I live without carbs?

The next report shows glycation's role in prostate cancer;

- **AGE/RAGE/AKT PATHWAY CONTRIBUTES TO PROSTATE CANCER CELL PROLIFERATION BY PROMOTING RB PHOSPHORYLATION AND DEGRADATION.**
"Metabolomic research has revealed that metabolites play an important role in prostate cancer development and progression. Previous studies have suggested that prostate cancer cell proliferation is induced by advanced glycation end products (AGEs) exposure, but the mechanism of this induction remains unknown. This study investigated the molecular mechanisms underlying the proliferative response of prostate cancer cell to the interaction of AGEs and the receptor for
advanced glycation end products (RAGE). To investigate this mechanism, we used Western blotting to evaluate the responses of the retinoblastoma (Rb), p-Rb and PI3K/Akt pathway to AGEs stimulation. We also examined the effect of knocking down Rb and blocking the PI3K/Akt pathway on AGEs

induced PC-3 cell proliferation. Our results indicated that AGE-RAGE interaction enhanced Rb phosphorylation and subsequently decreased total Rb levels. Bioinformatics analysis further indicated a negative correlation between RAGE and RB1 expression in prostate cancer tissue. Furthermore, we observed that AGEs stimulation activated the PI3K/Akt signaling pathway and that blocking PI3K/Akt signaling abrogated AGEs-induced cell proliferation. We report, for the first time, that AGE-RAGE interaction enhances prostate cancer cell proliferation by phosphorylation of Rb via the PI3K/Akt signaling pathway."

Published in Nov 2009, this report details the dangers of a carbohydrate diet, yet our industry has made sure that this report remained undisclosed. It's now 7 years later with over 315,000,000 more deaths from carb consumption occurring since then. Note the grammar used when referring to carbohydrate foods, they used the term *feeds* instead, implying livestock feed, when it's the carbohydrate foods that you eat that contribute to this disorder/disease. I wonder if this wording is due to influence from the food preparation industry (corporations selling the highest glycemic, most satiating foods on the market), which are backed by the industrialized farming industry, including companies like Monsanto, the leader in GMO crop seed, producing their GMO-Roundup ready seed specifically designed to withstand the enzyme changing properties in their glyphosate herbicide. I'm sure they didn't want this news being publicized, yet it was published in Nov 2009 at NIH's PubMed and nobody paid attention. I guess they were looking for their bagel. Were you ever told that a carbohydrate diet could do this damage? It makes me wonder, is Monsanto trying to hide what their crops do, to the people who consume them?

- ***HYPERGLYCEMIA IN CRITICAL ILLNESS: A REVIEW***
  "Hyperglycemia is commonplace in the critically ill patient and is associated with worse outcomes. It occurs after severe stress (e.g., infection or injury) and results from a combination of increased secretion of catabolic hormones, increased hepatic gluconeogenesis, and resistance to the peripheral and hepatic actions of insulin. The use of carbohydrate-based feeds, glucose-containing solutions, and drugs such as epinephrine may exacerbate the hyperglycemia. Mechanisms by which hyperglycemia cause harm are uncertain. Deranged osmolality and blood flow, intracellular acidosis, and enhanced superoxide production have all been implicated. The net result is a derangement of endothelial, immune and coagulation function and an association with neuropathy and myopathy. These changes can be prevented, at least in part, by the use of insulin to maintain normoglycemia."

YOU HAVE TWO CHOICES CONCERNING THIS GLUCOSE RUSE;
1. Continue the ruse by masturbating your taste buds and collect these diseases and disorders in return.
2. Stop taking part in it. Cut out as much as possible the starchy carbohydrates, and live free from dependence.

You need to realize that the comfort in comfort food, brings massive discomfort in the future, starting immediately, with a process called glycation. This is the real poisoning of America and we can correct it. It lies within our power, each and every one of us can correct this.

I offer a cure, not a therapy or treatment, My cure simply involves removal of all glycating substances from the diet to eliminate this problem of glycation so that it never affects the body. The glycating substances = carbs, sugar, glucose, fructose.

The above reports on the effects of glycation appeared in many cases, over 30 years ago in PubMed. I've shown you around 50 reports out of 11,750 studies to date detailing the damaging effects of Excessive Carbohydrate Consumption, the primary cause of glycation.

Why doesn't the FDA or the USDA say anything about that? The 42nd study, submitted in November 1989 shows how it causes inflammation, and with inflammation a factor in so many diseases, it truly is a wonder that the FDA and USDA never even issued anything so simple as a warning. The **FDA'S involvement in this matter is mostly explai**ned by their influence from the one industry, where they get most of their execs from, Monsanto.

From every form of cancer to Alzheimer's disease to heart disease and cardiovascular disease to arthritis to hypertension to high cholesterol these food sources (sugar and grains) are responsible for each and every one of these disorders. These studies are proof of exactly what sugar does to the body.

To cure the glycation factor in these diseases, the best way is to eliminate it as much as possible. To do that you must eliminate its source and to eliminate the source, you have to eliminate the grains and sugar.

In all, there were 3,629 studies in the fda's database on the effects of glucose glycating proteins, hemoglobin, and cholesterol dating back to march, 1984. Incidentally, that was one month after i was released from the hospital after spending a month in a coma and suffering two strokes while comatose. I could have never come back this far without dr. Perlmutter's help. Thank you, dr. Perlmutter.

With having the evidence for over 30 years, why hasn't the public been told about glycation or the ages they create? It's those ages that are at the root of all modern diseases. If this was uncovered 30+ years ago, why have we just found out about it from the bestselling books from two doctors? They were published in 2010 and 2012 and they had to dig this information out of the archives. Is someone trying to hide something? In whose best interest would it be to hide this information? The grain industry? My guess is yes.

The above reports on the effects of glycation appeared, in many cases, over 30 years ago in PubMed. With 11,667 studies to date detailing the damaging effects of Excessive Carbohydrate Consumption, the primary cause of glycation, why doesn't the FDA say anything? The last study, submitted in November 1989 shows how it causes inflammation and with inflammation a factor in so many diseases, it truly is a wonder that the FDA never even issued anything so simple as a warning. The **FDA's involvement** in this issue is mostly explained by their influence from the one industry where they get most of their execs from, Monsanto.

From every form of cancer to Alzheimer's disease to heart disease and cardiovascular disease to arthritis to hypertension to hyperlipidemia, these food sources (sugar and grains) are responsible for each and every one of these disorders. These studies are proof of exactly what sugar does to the body.

To cure the glycation factor in these diseases, the best way is to eliminate it as much as possible. To do that you must eliminate its source and to eliminate the source, you have to eliminate the grains and sugar that instigate it. Thank you, Dr. Davis and Dr. Perlmutter, for bringing this to my attention. It would have been nice if someone could have done it 20 or 30 years ago. For that, I thank the FDA, the USDA, and Monsanto. Don't allow them to be in your driver's seat. As long as you remain on your carbohydrate diet, they're in the driver's seat for your health. Give up the carbs and put yourself back in the driver's seat

COPIED FROM NOVA ON PBS
concerning Otzi, a 5,000-year-old frozen mummy;

" oeggl reconstructed the iceman's last meal from his microscopic analysis of a tiny sample removed from the mummy's transverse colon, the part of the intestine just beyond the stomach. When the iceman was discovered in 1991, x-rays and cat-scans of the corpse revealed that his internal organs had shrunken so drastically in the 5,300 years in the glacier that dr. Dieter zur nedden, the radiologist who examined the images, could barely distinguish them. Instead of filling the chest cavity with their billowy white form, the lungs looked like wisps of clouds.

But at the top of the colon, zur nedden made out a slight bulge, which the radiologist suspected was a clump of half-processed food. The progress of the food indicated that the iceman had last eaten about eight hours before he died, possibly of hypothermia, on the hauslabjoch pass, which cuts over the main alpine ridge dividing austria from italy at 10,500 feet above sea level.

Not until several years after the discovery did the innsbruck scientists finally cut a hole into the mummy, insert an endoscope, and snip out about .004 ounces from the colon. Dr. Werner platzer, the university of innsbruck anatomist then in charge of research on the corpse, gave .0016 ounces milligrams of the material to oeggl, who had already been studying the rich botanical finds from the site.

Pollen provided a snapshot of the environment the iceman was exposed to in the hours before his death oeggl 's sample was barely the size of his little fingernail. Under the microscope, he quickly identified the flake-like, semi-digested material that made up the bulk of the sample as einkorn, the most important wheat of the neolithic, the period of prehistory in which people lived in semi-permanent settlements and survived by agriculture and keeping animals. The discovery of einkorn, which does not occur naturally in europe, in the iceman's intestinal tract, suggested that he had contact with an agricultural community. The dominance of bran in the sample led oeggl to believe that the wheat had been finely ground into meal and made into bread, rather than eaten as a porridge, where the grains would have been eaten whole and found in larger pieces in the colon. But the bread would have been little like modern bread. In order to get bread to rise when yeast is added, the wheat grains must contain a high level of gluten, which lends the dough a durable elasticity and therefore holds the pockets of air. Einkorn has low levels of gluten, so the bread made with it, was probably hard, somewhat like a cracker, and rather tough on the teeth.

Using an electron microscope oeggl also spotted tiny particles of charcoal attached to the bran, probably remnants of the baking process on a hot rock, or next to a fire. In addition to the einkorn, the cells of at least one other plant, possibly some herb, were present in the sample, and oeggl concluded that they, too, had been part of his meal. He also found a tiny muscle fiber and a burned bit of bone, evidence that the iceman might also have eaten a meat. What kind of meat oeggl cannot *yet say, nor can he determine how much of the meal the sample represented.*

This feature originally appeared on the site for the nova program, *"Ice Mummies."* Although not shown in this excerpt, the iceman did show signs of modern day disease in his bones. It was evident mostly around his joints in the form of arthritis. This arthritis is directly due to his diet of einkorn wheat. As it does now, in glycating cholesterol it comes in contact with, it did so then. It just did it slower, due to the indigestibility of the einkorn wheat, but it occurred, never-the-less.

The damage it did at that time was much less than what it does now, due to the lack of fiber it has in today's strains of wheat, mostly the bread wheat made of **Triticum aestivum**, as well as Spelt, Durum, and Emmer. Even though arthritis seldom kills its victim, the damage it does, doesn't go away, ever. It's stuck to you like paint on a wall and you can't scrape it off. Most of today's wheat has, more tainted gluten protein than its ever had in its history, making it gluier and stickier, which makes it that much more dangerous, as this is what builds up more plaque in your system, and you already know what damage plaque does. This Einkorn wheat wasn't glyphosated, either. That, in itself, exponentially increases the inflammation that causes the arthritis and arthrosclerosis. If it's causing this, it's causing arteriosclerosis as well.

Perhaps the biggest question this brings up is, with all of this information available for this many years, why hasn't the FDA warned us that this food has these capabilities to do this kind of damage to the human body. Shouldn't the public be able to make an informed decision as to whether or not to continue to eat this food? Or should the FDA continue to ignore the evidence and fail to even let the public know what this food does? The question I want to ask, was there outside influence in their decision to not expose this information?

Someone is trying to keep this information unrevealed. They want to leave it up to an uneducated public to automatically know what these studies show. In whose best interest would it be to keep this information hidden? Whose business would hurt the most if bread and corn and wheat products all of a sudden became taboo? The grain industry? Monsanto? The more I look into this, the more it spells out cover-up and because this is how the FDA treats this, it instills a lot of fear in me as to how healthy the rest of our food supply is. The FDA has to know of the damage these grains do to the body when ingested, so why do they allow these industries to continue to peddle their wares as if they're healthy?

"Food, inc". Is a 2008 american **documentary film** directed by filmmaker **Robert Kenner**. The academy award-nominated film examines *corporate farming* in the *united states*, concluding that *agribusiness* produces *food that* is unhealthy, in a way that is environmentally harmful and abusive to both animals and employees. The film is narrated by **Michael Pollan** and **Eric Schlosser**. The film received positive responses and was nominated for several awards, including the *academy award* and the *independent spirit awards* in 2009, both for best documentary feature.

The film's first segment examines the industrial production of meat (chicken, beef, and pork), calling it inhumane and economically and environmentally **unsustainable**. The second segment looks at The **industrial production of grains and vegetables** (primarily corn and soybeans), again labeling this economically and environmentally unsustainable. The film's third and final segment is about the economic and legal power, such as **food labeling regulations**, of the major food companies, the profits of which are based on supplying cheap but contaminated food, the heavy use of petroleum-based chemicals (largely pesticides and fertilizers), and the promotion of unhealthy food consumption habits by the american public. This is a must see film, in my estimation, if you want to stay healthy.

EYE OPENING DOCUMENTARIES WELL WORTH WATCHING

Food, Inc	Overfed and Undernourished	Beyond our Differences
Food Beware		
Food Matters	**My Big Fat Body**	Why Are We Fat?
Food Choices	Facing the Fat	Is Sugar the New Fat?
Genetically Modified Foods	**Fat**	Sugar Blues
	Milk?	Shadows of Liberty
David vs Monsanto	**Fasting**	Circle of Poison
Of the Land	Food as Medicine	The Big Secret
Hungry for Change	**Beyond Food**	Supersized
That Sugar Film	Chemerical	Tricks of the Pharma Industry
Fathead	**Real Value**	
Heal Yourself	UnInflame Me	**Food as Medicine**
Love Paleo	**Sugar, the New Fat**	Fasting
Fresh	PurePlant Nation	

99

V

The Glyphosate Poisoning of America

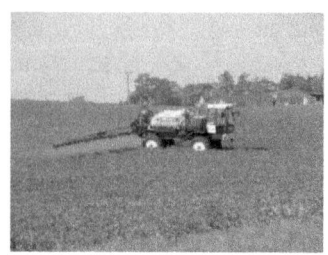

Monsanto's Covert Chemical Terrorism

Would you drink Roundup if you could? Probably not, at least, I wouldn't. Would you eat something that it's been doused in? If you knew that it was, you probably wouldn't touch that either. Do you realize that every bite of bread you take you're eating Roundup and substantial amounts of it, collectively? More than 1 million lbs of it are sprayed on crops every year, and you eat a good portion of that. Every corn chip you eat, you're eating unhealthy amounts of glyphosate with it. It's in the nature of how this herbicide is used. Do you drink soy milk? GMO soya was one of Monsanto's first GMO seeds, making it one the most heavily glyphosated grains, today. A large portion comes from Brazil where the glyphosate is killing farmers there, with cancer. It's also creating rivers out of farmland. Because of deforestation and growing soybeans, the water tables have risen. The roots of the forest went much deeper than the shallow roots of the soya plant, and the forest drank a lot more water than what the fields of soya use. This causes a rise in the water table. Due to this development, the higher water tables form underground rivers which are collapsing farmlands into above ground rivers.

The manifestation of this threat is directly due to your addiction to glucose, as that is the driving force that demands industry to accommodate this demand. That's why it's so important to curb the demand, by curbing the need, by breaking the addiction. Who knew that our greatest terrorist threat would be a clandestine threat from inside our country that doesn't carry a gun or bomb, or any kind of explosives, for that fact. This threat is a completely hidden threat, making it the worst threat we've ever faced. This threat is in your diet. It's in something you eat multiple times a day. In all actuality, your hunger cycle is the instrument of your destruction, with this threat. It's your hunger cycle that locks you into the cycle of destruction that glycation is responsible for as its the glucose that's responsible for all inflammation, which in turn, is responsible for all modern disease.

THIS IS THE THREAT OF THE GLUCOSE RUSE,

IT'S THE GLYPHOSATE THAT CATERS WHAT YOU'LL RUE,

BY CHEMICALLY CHANGING THE ENZYMES YOU USE,

WITH THE FOOD YOU EAT TO GIVE YOU THOSE BLUES.

All this damage from the enzyme inhibitors in the glyphosate, that's done to your hormones, is no small matter. These hormones are important hormones affecting digestion, hunger, fear, and sleep. (Those are the very same things affected by your diet. also.) Where's the similarity? It's explained in the way it affects its targeted enzymes, like tyrosine, tryptophan, and phenylalanine. These are all enzymes that influence your emotional, hunger, digestion and sleep hormones. If you have problems in any of these areas, this is your answer why. Because it affects your hunger, that proves it affects addiction, increasing it.

It involves your consumption of glyphosate. (I'll bet you didn't know that, did you?) Would you eat it in the first place, if you knew? You probably would because you've been addicted to what this substance has been sprayed on, without even knowing it. This was literally done right under your nose, when you were fed, as a baby. The industry makes certain that this substance gets into most all baby food. This ensures that you have no choice in this addiction. It ensures your lifetime of compliance in feeding the addiction. It also guarantees your compliance in the second half of the glucose ruse, the need for pharmaceuticals for a good portion of your life.

This is displayed in all the graphs below as the increase of glyphosate usage mirrors the increase in disease. Are you one of these statistics? If you eat bread, I'm afraid you are.

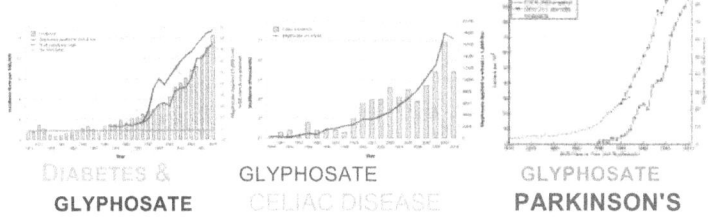

DIABETES &   GLYPHOSATE   GLYPHOSATE
GLYPHOSATE   CELIAC DISEASE   **PARKINSON'S**

In the next chapter, you'll see a graph like these for phobias and glyphosate, showing how it's increased our fear levels, as a nation of glyphosate consumers.

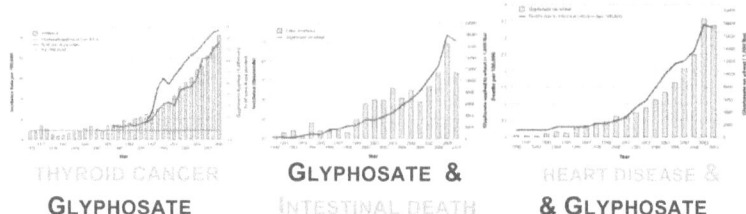

| Thyroid Cancer & Glyphosate | Glyphosate & Intestinal Death | Heart Disease & Glyphosate |

Because of its importance, I repeat, another graph for phobias and glyphosate shows the same increase. Your fears increased by glyphosate consumption. (You'll see the importance of this in the next chapter.) Targeted enzymes that influence the senescence of plants also influence the senescence of your body. These important enzymes are enzymes your body uses for digestion and controlling hunger, and they are altered in their function by glyphosate. The chemicals imported into your system by your diet are altering your enzymatic ability to fully digest your food, control your emotions, and get your proper sleep. Do you use Ambien or Prozac?

"Serotonin (a neurotransmitter), synthesized by tryptophan hydroxylase, Melatonin (a neurohormone) is in turn synthesized from serotonin, via N-acetyltransferase and 5-hydroxyindole-O-methyltransferase enzymes. Niacin, also known as vitamin B_3, is synthesized from tryptophan via kynurenine and quinolinic acids."

"Entropy is a monthly peer-reviewed open access scientific journal covering research on all aspects of entropy and information theory. It was established in 1999 and is published by MDPI. The journal regularly publishes special issues compiled by guest editors.[1] The editor-in-chief is Kevin H. Knuth (University at Albany, SUNY)".

In 2013, Entropy published a review paper saying glyphosate may be the most important factor in the development of obesity, depression, attention deficit hyperactivity disorder, autism, Alzheimer's disease, Parkinson's disease, multiple sclerosis, cancer, and infertility.

As explained in Wikipedia:
Amino acids, including tryptophan, are used as building blocks in protein biosynthesis, and proteins are required to sustain life. Many animals (including humans) cannot synthesize tryptophan:

they need to obtain it through their diet, making it an essential amino acid. Tryptophan is among the less common amino acids found in proteins, but it plays important structural or functional roles whenever it occurs. For instance, tryptophan and tyrosine residues play special roles in "anchoring" membrane proteins within the cell membrane. In addition, tryptophan functions as a biochemical precursor for the following compounds

In November 2015, the European Food Safety Authority published an updated assessment report on glyphosate, concluding that "the substance is unlikely to be genotoxic (i.e. damaging to DNA) or to pose a carcinogenic threat to humans.

- " Furthermore, the final report clarified that while other, probably carcinogenic, glyphosate-containing formulations may exist, studies "that look solely at the active substance glyphosate do not show this effect. In May 2016, the Joint FAO/WHO Meeting on Pesticide Residues concluded that "glyphosate is unlikely to pose a carcinogenic risk to humans from exposure through the diet, even at doses as high as 2,000 mg/kg body weight orally. " I have to question their judgment. I don't believe they're looking at all the aspects of glyphosate and how enzyme rearrangement does cause derangement. They're obviously not looking at the graphs of the diseases alongside the graphs of the glyphosate spraying. They clearly show the devastation this herbicide has wrought.
These targeted enzymes are important for digestion, hunger, and sleep.
- *Tyrosine influences hunger by controlling enzymes that control how receptors react to stimuli that control your hunger. Tyrosine is a precursor to Dopamine, your primary hormone influencing hunger. This is the hormone triggered by leptin, your satiety hormone. If it takes more leptin to trigger the dopamine, it's going to take more food to trigger the leptin.* Was this engineered intentionally?
- *Tryptophan is also a precursor to serotonin and melatonin. Serotonin is another feel-good hormone that's affected by glyphosate. Melatonin is the hormone that allows you to sleep. without it, you're going to have trouble sleeping.* Is it no wonder why so many people suffer from insomnia now? Ambien anyone?
- *Phenylalanine is a precursor to tyrosine; the monoamine neurotransmitters dopamine, norepinephrine (noradrenaline), and epinephrine (adrenaline); and the skin pigment melanin.* All these enzymes influence your hunger and energy.

Recent studies have produced tumors, the relative size of boulders, in the abdomens of rats, administered what's considered "safe dosages". The videos of these rats is thoroughly disgusting. But, they're opening eyes.

The WHO has finally recognized glyphosate as a **GROUP 2 CARCINOGEN**, meaning that it probably causes cancer. We know that it affects your sleep, hunger, and digestion, let's see if these chemicals can be responsible for cancer. The evidence for this lies in the multiple graphs showing the increase of glyphosate increasing right alongside the increase of multiple disorders and disease, including autism.

Monsanto's Glyphosate Ruse

In Monsanto's desire to spread as much of this on the earth as possible, they're poisoning every bit of food you eat, unless you grow your own food, and raise and butcher your own meat. All forage for feed is sprayed multiple times, maybe even more than the grain used for your bread. Cattle slaughtered for beef, never live long enough to get cancer, yet it goes into their food supply. 1.8 billion lbs in 20 years have been dumped on your food supplies. Ultimately, it goes into your body in multiple avenues, increasing the amount you consume, thereby increasing the amount of enzyme inhibitors affecting your health. This has brought the pharmaceutical industry record profits, not to mention what it's brought Monsanto and their crop seed companies, pharmaceutical companies, and the chemical wing of their manufacturing. Monsanto has engineered clandestine distemper on our health without us even knowing or approving of it.

- **_Glyphosate, pathways to modern diseases III: Manganese, neurological diseases, and associated pathologies_**

  Glyphosate is a likely cause of the recent epidemic in celiac disease. Glyphosate residues are found in wheat due to the increasingly widespread practice of staging and desiccation of wheat right before harvest. Many of the pathologies associated with celiac disease can be explained by disruption of CYP enzymes. Celiac patients have a shortened life span, mainly due to an increased risk of cancer, most especially non-Hodgkin's lymphoma, which has also been linked to glyphosate. Celiac disease trends over time match well with the increase in glyphosate usage on wheat crops.

  Glyphosate is also neurotoxic. Its mammalian metabolism yields two products: Aminomethylphosphonic acid (AMPA) and glyoxylate, with AMPA being at least as toxic as glyphosate. Glyoxylate is a highly reactive glycating agent, which will disrupt the function of multiple proteins in cells that are exposed. Glycation has been directly implicated in Parkinson's disease (PD). Glyphosate has been detected in the brains of malformed piglets. In a report produced by the Environmental Protection Agency (EPA), over 36% of 271 incidences involving acute glyphosate poisoning involved neurological symptoms, indicative of glyphosate toxicity in the brain and nervous system.

In the remainder of this paper, we first introduce the link between glyphosate and manganese (Mn) dysbiosis and briefly describe the main biological roles of Mn. We then describe how glyphosate's disruption of gut bacteria may be a major player in the recent epidemic in antibiotic resistance. We then explain how glyphosate can influence the uptake of arsenic and aluminum, and propose similar mechanisms at work with Mn. In the next section, we describe how Mn deficiency can lead to a reduction in Lactobacillus in the gut, and we link this to anxiety disorder. We follow with a discussion on mitochondrial dysfunction associated with suppressed Mn superoxide dismutase (Mn-SOD), and then a section on implications of Mn deficiency for oxalate metabolism. The following section explains how Mn deficiency can lead to the overexpression of ammonia and glutamate in many neurological diseases. The next two sections show how Mn accumulation in the liver is linked to cholestasis and high serum low-density lipoprotein (LDL), and how this can also induce increased susceptibility to Salmonella poisoning. We then identify a role for Mn in chondroitin sulfate synthesis and the implications for osteomalacia. The next two sections explain how glyphosate exposure can lead to Mn toxicity in the brain, and discuss two neurological diseases that are associated with excess Mn, PD and prion diseases. After a section on the link between male infertility and Mn deficiency in the testes, we discuss evidence of exposure to glyphosate and end with a short summary of our findings.

The report goes on to detail how this herbicide is involved in suppressing dopamine which leads to an overactive thyroid. It's also involved in ;

1. **MICROBIAL ANTIBIOTIC INTOLERANCE**
    Manganese (Mn) is an often overlooked but important nutrient, required in small amounts for multiple essential functions in the body. A recent study on cows fed genetically modified Roundup®-Ready feed revealed a severe depletion of serum Mn. Glyphosate, the active ingredient in Roundup®, has also been shown to severely deplete Mn levels in plants. Here, we investigate the impact of Mn on physiology, and its association with gut dysbiosis as well as neuropathologies such as autism,

Alzheimer's disease (AD), depression, anxiety syndrome, Parkinson's disease (PD), and prion diseases. Glutamate overexpression in the brain in association with autism, AD, and other neurological diseases can be explained by Mn deficiency. Mn superoxide dismutase protects mitochondria from oxidative damage, and mitochondrial dysfunction is a key feature of autism and Alzheimer's. Chondroitin sulfate synthesis depends on Mn, and its deficiency leads to osteoporosis and osteomalacia. Lactobacillus, depleted in autism, depend critically on Mn for antioxidant protection. Lactobacillus probiotics can treat anxiety, which is a comorbidity of autism and chronic fatigue syndrome. Reduced gut Lactobacillus leads to overgrowth of the pathogen, Salmonella, which is resistant to glyphosate toxicity, and Mn plays a role here as well. Sperm motility depends on Mn, and this may partially explain increased rates of infertility and birth defects. We further reason that, under conditions of adequate Mn in the diet, glyphosate, through its disruption of bile acid homeostasis, ironically promotes toxic accumulation of Mn in the brainstem, leading to conditions such as PD and prion diseases.

2. **MANGANESE DYSBIOSIS DUE TO GLYPHOSATE**

    Remarkably, Mn deficiency can explain many of the pathologies associated with autism and Alzheimer's disease (AD). The incidence of both of these conditions has been increasing at an alarming rate in the past two decades, in step with the increased usage of glyphosate on corn and soy crops in the United States.

3. **ANALOGY WITH ARSENIC AND ALUMINUM**

    Chronic kidney disease is clearly associated with multiple environmental toxicants. There has been an epidemic in recent years in kidney failure among young agricultural workers in Central America, India, and Sri Lanka, particularly those working in the sugar cane fields. A recent paper reached the unmistakable conclusion that glyphosate plays a critical role in this epidemic. A growing practice of spraying sugar cane with glyphosate as a ripener and desiccant right before the harvest has led to much greater exposure to the workers in the fields. The authors, who focused their studies on affected workers in rice paddies in Sri Lanka, identified a synergistic effect of arsenic, which contaminated the soil in the affected regions. This paper is highly significant because it proposes a mechanism whereby glyphosate greatly increases the toxicity of arsenic through chelation, which promotes uptake by the gut. Glyphosate also depletes glutathione (GSH) and glutathione S transferase (GST) is a critical enzyme for liver detoxification of arsenic. As a consequence, excess arsenic in the kidney

causes acute kidney failure, without evidence of other symptoms such as diabetes usually preceding kidney failure.
4. **ANALOGY WITH ARSENIC AND ALUMINUM**
5. **MN-SUPEROXIDE DISMUTASE & MITOCHONDRIAL DYSFUNCTION**
6. **GUT BACTERIA DYSBIOSIS AND ANXIETY**
7. **AMMONIA, GLUTAMATE, AND NEUROTOXICITY**

In this section, we will show that both glutamate and ammonia are implicated as neurotoxins in connection with autism and other neurological diseases, and we will offer the simple explanation that Mn deficiency leads to impaired activity of glutamine synthase and arginase, both of which utilize Mn as a cofactor. Mn deficiency can also explain the increased risk of epilepsy found in autism, due to the fact that Mn decreases T2 relaxation time. Mn-deprived rats are more susceptible to convulsions.

Many diseases and conditions are currently on the rise in step with glyphosate usage in agriculture, particularly on GM crops of corn and soy. These include autism, AD, PD, anxiety disorder, osteoporosis, inflammatory bowel disease, renal lithiasis, osteomalacia, cholestasis, thyroid dysfunction, and infertility. All of these conditions can be substantially explained by the dysregulation of Mn utilization in the body due to glyphosate.

It may seem implausible that glyphosate could be toxic to humans, given the fact that government regulators appear nonchalant about steadily increasing residue limits, and that the levels in food and water are rarely monitored by government agencies, presumably due to lack of concern. However, a paper by Antoniou ET AL. provided a scathing indictment of the European regulatory process regarding glyphosate's toxicity, focusing on potential teratogenic effects. They identified several key factors leading to a tendency to overlook potential toxic effects. These include using animal studies that are too short or have too few animals to achieve statistical significance, disregarding IN VITRO studies or studies with exposures that are higher than what is expected to be realistically present in food, and discarding studies that examine the effects of glyphosate formulations rather than pure glyphosate, even though formulations are a more realistic model of the natural setting and are often orders of magnitude more toxic than the active ingredient in pesticides. Regulators also seemed unaware that chemicals that act as endocrine disruptors (such as glyphosate often have an inverted dose-response relationship, wherein very low doses can have more acute effects than higher doses. Teratogenic effects have been demonstrated in human cell lines. An IN VITRO study showed that glyphosate in parts per trillion can induce human breast cancer cell proliferation.

8. PARKINSON'S DISEASE
9. PRION DISEASES
10. OSTEOMALACIA AND ARTHRITIS

This is only a partial list of what this herbicide is responsible for. This just points out the fact that what you eat has more impact on your health than anything else. It would be nice if you could get away from it, but you can't. The pollution is everywhere you go for food. You have to produce your own food to be completely free from this curse.

It's cursing you not only through the grains you eat but through the damage done to feed crops, contaminating beef, pork, chicken, turkey and even dairy cows, poisoning even the cheese, milk and butter you buy. The only way you can get around this ruse is to grow your own food and raise and butcher your own meat. Monsanto has every other path sewn up, tighter than a drum. To eat grains is to court death. It's become that simple.

- ***Glyphosate, pathways to modern diseases II: Celiac sprue and gluten intolerance***
  Celiac disease, and, more generally, gluten intolerance, is a growing problem worldwide, but especially in North America and Europe, where an estimated 5% of the population now suffers from it. Symptoms include nausea, diarrhea, skin rashes, macrocytic anemia, and depression. It is a multifactorial disease associated with numerous nutritional deficiencies as well as reproductive issues and increased risk of thyroid disease, kidney failure, and cancer. Here, we propose that glyphosate, the active ingredient in the herbicide, Roundup®, is the most important causal factor in this epidemic. Fish exposed to glyphosate develop digestive problems that are reminiscent of celiac disease. Celiac disease is associated with imbalances in gut bacteria that can be fully explained by the known effects of glyphosate on gut bacteria. Characteristics of celiac disease point to impairment in many cytochrome P450 enzymes, which are involved with detoxifying environmental toxins, activating vitamin D3, catabolizing vitamin A, and maintaining bile acid production and sulfate supplies to the gut. Glyphosate is known to inhibit cytochrome P450 enzymes. Deficiencies in iron, cobalt, molybdenum, copper and other rare metals associated with celiac disease can be attributed to glyphosate's strong ability to chelate these elements. Deficiencies in tryptophan, tyrosine, methionine, and selenomethionine associated with celiac disease match glyphosate's known depletion of these amino acids. Celiac disease patients have an increased risk to non-Hodgkin's lymphoma, which has also been implicated in glyphosate exposure. Reproductive issues associated with celiac disease, such as infertility,

miscarriages, and birth defects, can also be explained by glyphosate. Glyphosate residues in wheat and other crops are likely increasing recently due to the growing practice of crop desiccation just prior to the harvest. We argue that the practice of "ripening" sugar cane with glyphosate may explain the recent surge in kidney failure among agricultural workers in Central America. We conclude with a plea to governments to reconsider policies regarding the safety of glyphosate residues in foods.

Gut bacteria

We then show that glyphosate is associated with an overgrowth of pathogens along with an inflammatory bowel disease in animal models. A parallel exists with celiac disease where the bacteria that are positively and negatively affected by glyphosate are overgrown or underrepresented respectively in association with celiac disease in humans.

- *CYP Enzyme impairment and sulfate depletion*
- *Retinoic acid, celiac disease, and reproductive issues*
- *Anemia and iron*

  Glyphosate's chelating action can have profound effects on iron in plants (Eker ET AL., 2006; Bellaloui ET AL., 2009). Glyphosate interferes with iron assimilation in both glyphosate-resistant and glyphosate-sensitive soybean crops (Bellaloui ET AL., 2009). It is therefore conceivable that glyphosate's chelation of iron is responsible for the refractory iron deficiency present in celiac disease.

- *Molybdenum deficiency*
- *Selenium and thyroid disorders*
- *Indole and kidney disease*
- *Nutritional deficiencies*

  Glyphosate disrupts the synthesis of tryptophan and tyrosine in plants and in gut bacteria, due to its interference with the shikimate pathway (Lu ET AL., 2013; María ET AL., 1996), which is its main source of toxicity to plants. Glyphosate also depletes methionine in plants and microbes. A study on serum tryptophan levels in children with celiac disease revealed that untreated children had significantly lower ratios of tryptophan to large neutral amino acids in the blood, and treated children also had lower levels, but the imbalance was less severe (Hernanz & Polanco, 1991).

- *Cancer*

"Chronic inflammation, such as occurs in celiac disease, is a major source of oxidative stress and is estimated to account for 1/3 of all cancer cases worldwide Oxidative stress leads to DNA damage and increased risk to genetic mutation. Several population-based studies have confirmed that patients with celiac disease suffer from increased mortality, mainly due to malignancy These include increased risk to non-Hodgkin's lymphoma, adenocarcinoma of the small intestine, and squamous cell carcinomas of the esophagus, mouth, and pharynx, as well as melanoma. The non-Hodgkin's lymphoma was not restricted to gastrointestinal sites, and the increased risk remained following a gluten-free diet "

Evidence of cancer rising in farm workers that have to work with this chemical.

- **_Proposed transglutaminase-glyphosate interactions_**
- **_Evidence of glyphosate exposure in humans and animals_**
- **_Kidney disease in agricultural workers_**

"In another study in the PMC database of over 164 studies done on this subject; Celiac disease, and, more generally, gluten intolerance, is a growing problem worldwide, but especially in North America and Europe, where an estimated 5% of the population now suffers from it. Symptoms include nausea, diarrhea, skin rashes, macrocytic anemia, and depression. It is a multifactorial disease associated with numerous nutritional deficiencies as well as reproductive issues and increased risk to thyroid disease, kidney failure and cancer. Here, we propose that glyphosate, the active ingredient in the herbicide, Roundup®, is the most important causal factor in this epidemic. Fish exposed to glyphosate develop digestive problems that are reminiscent of celiac disease. Celiac disease is associated with imbalances in gut bacteria that can be fully explained by the known effects of glyphosate on gut bacteria. Characteristics of celiac disease point to impairment in many cytochrome P450 enzymes, which are involved with detoxifying environmental toxins, activating vitamin D3, catabolizing vitamin A, and maintaining bile acid production and sulfate supplies to the gut. Glyphosate is known to inhibit cytochrome P450 enzymes. Deficiencies in iron, cobalt, molybdenum, copper and other rare metals associated with celiac disease can be attributed to glyphosate's strong ability to chelate these elements.

Deficiencies in tryptophan, tyrosine, methionine, and selenomethionine associated with celiac disease match glyphosate's known depletion of these amino acids. Celiac disease patients have an increased risk to non-Hodgkin's lymphoma, which has also been implicated in glyphosate exposure. Reproductive issues associated with celiac disease, such as infertility, miscarriages, and birth defects, can also be explained by glyphosate. Glyphosate residues in wheat and other crops are likely increasing recently due to the growing practice of crop desiccation just prior to the harvest. We argue that the practice of "ripening" sugar cane with glyphosate may explain the recent surge in kidney failure among agricultural workers in Central America. We conclude with a plea to governments to reconsider policies regarding the safety of glyphosate residues in foods."

- **Republished study: long-term toxicity of a Roundup herbicide and a Roundup-tolerant genetically modified maize**
  Biochemical analyses confirmed very significant chronic kidney deficiencies, for all treatments and both sexes; 76% of the altered parameters were kidney-related. In treated males, liver congestions and necrosis were 2.5 to 5.5 times higher. Marked and severe nephropathies were also generally 1.3 to 2.3 times greater. In females, all treatment groups showed a two- to threefold increase in mortality, and deaths were earlier. This difference was also evident in three male groups fed with GM maize. All results were hormone- and sex-dependent, and the pathological profiles were comparable. Females developed large mammary tumors more frequently and before controls; the pituitary was the second most disabled organ; the sex hormonal balance was modified by consumption of GM maize and Roundup treatments. Males presented up to four times more large palpable tumors starting 600 days earlier than in the control group, in which only one tumor was noted. These results may be explained by not only the non-linear endocrine-disrupting effects of Roundup but also by the overexpression of the EPSPS transgene or other mutational effects in the GM maize and their metabolic consequences.
  Our findings show that the differences in multiple organ functional parameters seen from the consumption of NK603 GM maize for 90 days escalated over 2 years into severe organ damage in all types of test diets. This included the lowest dose

of R administered (0.1 ppb, 50 ng/L G equivalent) of R formulation administered, which is well below permitted MRLs in both the USA (0.7 mg/L) and European Union (100 ng/L). Surprisingly, there was also a clear trend in increased tumor incidence, especially mammary tumors in female animals, in a number of the treatment groups. Our data highlight the inadequacy of 90-day feeding studies and the need to conduct long-term (2 years) investigations to evaluate the life-long impact of GM food consumption and exposure to complete pesticide formulations.

Tumors are reported in line with the requirements of OECD chronic toxicity protocols 452 and 453, which require all 'lesions' (which by definition include tumors) to be reported. These findings are summarized in Figure 4. The results are presented in the form of real-time cumulative curves (each step corresponds to an additional tumor in the group). Only the growing largest palpable growths (above a diameter of 17.5 mm in females and 20 mm in males) are presented (for example, see Figure 5A, B, C). These were found to be in 95% of cases non-regressive tumors (Figure 5D, E, F, G, H, I, J) and were not infectious nodules. These arose from time to time; then, most often disappeared and were not different from controls after bacterial analyses. The real tumors were recorded independently of their grade, but dependent on their morbidity, since non-cancerous tumors can be more lethal than those of cancerous nature, due to internal hemorrhaging or compression and obstruction of the function of vital organs, or toxins or hormone secretions. These tumors progressively increased in size and number, but not proportionally to the treatment dose, over the course of the experiment (Figure 4). As in the case of rates of mortality (Figure 6), this suggests that a threshold in effect was reached at the lower doses. Tumor numbers were rarely equal but almost always more than in controls for all treated groups, often with a two- to threefold increase for both sexes. Tumors began to reach a large size on average 94 days before controls in treated females and up to 600 days earlier in two male groups fed with GM maize (11 and 22% with or without R).

- **_Glyphosate formulations induce apoptosis and necrosis in human umbilical, embryonic, and placental cells._**

  We have evaluated the toxicity of four glyphosate (G)-based herbicides in Roundup formulations, from 10(5) times dilutions, on three different human cell types. This dilution level is far below agricultural recommendations and corresponds to low levels of residues in food or feed. The formulations have been compared to G alone and with its main metabolite AMPA or *with one known adjuvant of R formulations, POEA. HUVEC primary neonate umbilical cord vein cells have been tested with 293 embryonic kidney and JEG3 placental cell lines. All R formulations cause total cell death within 24 h, through an inhibition of the mitochondrial succinate dehydrogenase activity, and necrosis, by the release of cytosolic adenylate kinase measuring membrane damage. They also induce apoptosis via activation of enzymatic caspases 3/7 activity. This is confirmed by characteristic DNA fragmentation, nuclear shrinkage (pyknosis), and nuclear fragmentation (karyorrhexis), which is demonstrated by DAPI in apoptotic round cells. G provokes only apoptosis, and HUVEC are 100 times more sensitive overall at this level. The deleterious effects are not proportional to G concentrations but rather depend on the nature of the adjuvants. AMPA and POEA separately and synergistically damage cell membranes like R but at different concentrations. Their mixtures are generally even more harmful with G. In conclusion, the R adjuvants like POEA change human cell permeability and amplify toxicity induced already by G, through apoptosis and necrosis. The real threshold of G toxicity must take into account the presence of adjuvants but also G metabolism and time-amplified effects or bioaccumulation. This should be discussed when analyzing the in vivo toxic actions of R. This work clearly confirms that the adjuvants in Roundup formulations are not inert. Moreover, the proprietary mixtures available on the market could cause cell damage and even death around residual levels to be expected, especially in food and feed derived from R formulation-treated crops.*

This poses a major question in my mind; can the target in this ruse, be you and your money? It's obvious what the end result is and that's displayed in the record profits of the pharmaceutical industry. The more disease caused by this herbicide, the more medicine the pharmaceutical industry sells. Monsanto owns the crop seed companies, produces the herbicide and owns the pharmaceutical corporations, so they're profiting much more than two or three times in this ruse. It's that simple. Only you can control this this travesty of justice, this transformation of your health. Only you can say no to the grains that this herbicide poisons. It's your choice to remain a slave to Monsanto or be free. All you have to do is to give up the grains.

VI

The Real Reason Terrorism Exists and Thrives

Our Addiction to Sugar and its True Costs

This is why we are an obese, diabetic, diseased society stricken with fear, anger, and terrorism all driven by an incessant hunger driven by corporate America responsible for our food supply. These are the same people who sell us all of our medicines. What makes you sick? To answer that question with all full honesty, you must first ask yourself, what makes you hungry? I can answer that question in 3 words, what you eat. If you're eating food that makes you sick, you get amazingly well when you stop eating it. (That's exactly what happened to me.)

This can be summed with one word, ADDICTION. Only addiction can make a person sick when they can't get their addiction fed or when that addiction affects other functions in the body. Only a societal addiction can drive a society to act and react like our spedies has been doing for the last 8,000 years. You may think I'm crazy, but I'm going to tell you just why I think this way. I'll give you evidence of why I think like this and let you be the judge. As a species, we started cultivating wheat for just about as far back as 8-10,000 years. The Hebrew bible, which dates to 10,000 BCE has scriptures of bread being part of the diet of Abraham, in the Book of Genesis.

For me, it started 5 years ago when I was trying to lose weight past a certain point that I couldn't get past, even though I was exercising 4-5 times a week for 3-4 hours each time, and not losing anything. I decided it had to do with what I was eating and sure enough, as soon as I gave up the bread, my weight started disappearing. (What was made from wheat, I didn't eat.) I felt so great just after giving up the bread that I decided to give up all grains....even my precious steel cut oats. (For the extent of my life, I thought that oatmeal was supposed to be good for you). After I gave up all grains I lost more weight, lost more pain, had fewer headaches, as they'd almost become a thing of the past at this point. I then decided to give up all carbs. That was a tough decision. I wrestled with it for weeks, before I did, but when I did finally "take the leap", my whole life changed like I never anticipated.

I learned that the one food that I had been encouraged to eat my whole life, was the one food that was tearing down my body while it was wearing down my brain. This is the food that's been making me sick. And I thought it was supposed to be good for me. I, like you, had been duped. I've learned over the last 5 years, that our bodies survive much better without any kind of carb intrusion at all.

I've learned in the last 4 years, why the digestion of carbs and sugar create virtually all disease. I learned in the last 2 years that that action of why carbs drag us down so much, (glycation), has been magnified by multiple applications of a glyphosate pesticide that inhibits enzymes, in the nature of how it kills weeds.

It's also killing massive amounts of people. It's easy to see, that the increase in the frequency of occurrence, the increased severity, and in the number of cases reported of all modern major diseases, follow the same graph lines as the usage of glyphosate pesticides sprayed on all GMO crops. (over 900 million lbs a year is sprayed.) Isn't industrial farming something to behold? Maybe for the investor but not for the farmer, consumer, or the public at large. For them, it's much more than that, it's costly emotionally, financially and physically. It's costly to the point of taking their life. it's downright deadly. Just ask Senator John McCain about his glioblastoma (brain cancer). That's what took my niece 25 years ago. I recently met a new friend who's suffered severely, to the point of near death, from her exposure to glyphosate, sprayed on fields in Yuma, AZ.

Monsanto can continue to deny that their pesticide *Roundup* was ever dangerous, but they won't be able to much longer. Lawsuits are already starting to stack up in the courthouses, with farmers and crop-dusters suing Monsanto for cancer they've gotten just from handling the chemicals. Think how a lifetime of consumption is going to affect one's health. Little by little, it eats away at your health by changing the way your enzymes work. This is Monsanto's gift to mankind. I guess it's their idea of "better living through chemistry." What was it Stalin said? "Control the food, control the people." Is Monsanto heeding this? Remember the graphs from chapter 5, *The Glyphosate Poisoning of America?* Here's the graph for phobias and glyphosate. That means if you're more afraid, today, than you were ten years ago, this is why and it also means that you will be, more so, ten years from now, but only if you keep eating their weed killer. Do you listen to the President, to fear what he fears?

With fear begetting hate, anger, antagonism, violence, and terrorism, it's definitely not my idea of better living, and this is why I blame a good portion of the woes of society, today, on this industry. Would you call this better living. through chemistry?

But it's not completely their responsibility either. It's the fault of misplaced trust in gov't agencies to keep us safe by what they recommend for us to eat. We did, after all, have to fall into this pit. The USDA, for example, tells us what to put on our plate according to what the farmer can grow the most of and not what's healthy to eat. It's really pretty simple. They won't recommend what's safe to eat due to Monsanto's industrial farming control and the fact that many department. heads and directors in the USDA, FDA, and even probably the EPA, came directly, or indirectly from Monsanto. And, we mindlessly allow that control without any vetting of it, on our own. (But then, how are we supposed to know where to investigate?) That, combined with the control they have over the pharmaceutical industry. They've politically engineered the control of America, through their food. They took Stalin's words to heart, to destroy our hearts.

The problem here is that Monsanto owns a majority of farmers in America by having them all contracted to grow their GMO wheat, sugar cane, corn, soy, oats, rice, potatoes, cotton, and a whole lot more. They virtually ended the seed-cleaning business in Indiana, simply to sell more of their GMO seed to more farmers, so they could sell more *Roundup*. Seed cleaning used to be a thriving business in farming communities. They made their money from cleaning a certain portion of a farmer's crop to give him back seed to plant next year. This was how genetic engineering took place for hundreds of years. The farmer would choose the best yielding portion of his field to clean for next year's seed. But, since Monsanto has patented genetic engineering of plants and seeds, now, it's a whole different story. Ender seeds have taken over the industry, limiting all crops to GMO, if their industrially grown. All fast food is industrially grown making it some of the highest glyphosated food you can eat. More on this coming up in chapter 8.

Now, genetic engineering means, to modify plants to accept *Roundup* herbicide and still live. This delivers the chemicals into the food you eat, to change your hormones, due to its prevalence in all grains, including sugar. Even GMO-free sugar can be affected. How do you know the sugar in your danish, this morning had no glyphosate in it? You don't, and that's the problem. (More on that in Chapter 8, *The Restaurant Ruse of the Glucose Ruse*.)

What used to be a family venture, running the farm, is now an industrial venture, almost completely corporate controlled. We just learned how corporations, control things. They have to control things for the bottom line only, in many cases. Their shareholders demand it. So they're forced to hurt, injure and harm their consumers all for the sake of increasing shareholder returns. That's the law of capitalism where gain or profit, not health, is the bottom line.

This is the nature of corporate control, to control a market to the extent that you find multiple avenues of income through your extensive control. This is why they sell the same chemicals to Pfizer. Pfizer used to be a part of Monsanto before it became Pfizer. It was Pharmacia, then, and they sell the same drugs now, that they sold, then. Monsanto provides them with the same chemicals that they douse their crops with to put in their medicines. (Their chemicals are everywhere, literally).

With its placements of directors, lawyers and lobbyists in the halls of the USDA, FDA, EPA and maybe even the CDC, Monsanto has pretty much taken over control of these agencies. All of these agencies that are supposed to be regulating Monsanto's industries and companies, seem to be as impotent as a castrata in a 19th century Viennese choir. Because Monsanto pretty much controls what the USDA says, they've aimed our society in a direction that can only lead us to the brink of disaster by making and keeping everybody sick, hungry, in fear, and worse yet even more addicted than they were when they were born. Yeah, this is an addiction that everyone has, as everyone was born into it. These industries use this addiction to take your money multiple times.

Actually, you pay this industry more than any other entity. When you buy groceries, you're paying this industry. When you buy medicine for the pain that their food creates, you're paying this industry. When they ultimately hospitalize you for heart disease or cancer or Alzheimer's disease, you'll be paying them again. You'll forever be in their hold once you start on their medications. From then on, it's all downhill into an abyss of pain, misery, and lingering death.

It's the USDA that recommends what to put on your plate to eat. Pretty much every other agency follows suit and recommends the same food. Why? This is food that Monsanto grows. They grow it through their contracted farmers all growing their glyphosate ready seed that they will spray the chemicals on, multiple times. And yes, this does eventually make you sick, if you eat it, but only if you eat it. Although, I do fear groundwater contamination. With the spraying so prevalent, groundwater is getting contaminated, now. Bees and butterflies are also dying due to glyphosate spraying. But that's another story. We're talking about what the *Roundup* does to our bodies and why they can do it, right now. It's because what they sell as food, is addictive, to begin with.

Monsanto uses that against us. They know our society is addicted. They've worsened it, by far. They've taken our addiction and turned it to their favor by ramping it up. This increases the need for the pharmaceuticals Pfizer sells. Do you smell a rat? I smell a Glucose Ruse. The biggest and by far, worst joke ever to be played on mankind. What Monsanto has done is create a world of anger, animosity, and antagonism by playing our emotions against our hunger. Our President is a shining example of the fear that extreme carbolism creates. Only fear could drive him to do the things he's apparently done throughout his life to get where he's gotten. Because of his addiction, everything in his brain is deranged. You can see the derangement in his body and in his demeanor.

Because of our addiction, everything in our bodies and brains is deranged. Everything. I know. I gave up the carbs and learned the truth. You'd have to give them up also, to fully know the truth. You may have suspected this for a while, but you'll never know the real truth until you break the addiction that you were born with. Once you break this addiction a whole new world opens up, mostly due to the mental clarity you gain without the grains. But, also due to the increase in energy you'll experience. The longer you stay away from carbs, the more energy you get and the more intelligent you get, and the healthier you ultimately get. Illnesses will become a thing of the past, but you have to give up the carbs for this to happen.

I blame our current state of affairs on a Supreme Court decision that gives corporations the same rights as individuals, even though they don't have the same moral compass, nor do they always adhere to the law. How do you put a corporation in jail for murder? You can't. You can only fine them, which is written off as an expense. And then, deducted from taxes, as an expense. (It just creative bookkeeping and it's only illegal if you get caught, as our President has just shown.)

How can you hold a corporation accountable for genocide? Monsanto's glyphosate *Roundup* and pesticides are directly responsible for more deaths in the last 40 years than any other single cause. The Glucose Ruse that they'd perpetrated has and is responsible for over 2000 deaths every day in America, alone. Imagine what it is around the whole world? Now that glyphosate has been generically made since the patent expired in 2000, it's even more prevalent.

Our Supreme Court has basically given their approval to this when they agreed to allow all corporations to have the same rights as a person who has to live by the law. We know how much corporations skirt the law. They have to. Their bylaws tell them to take all steps necessary to increase profits and boost the investment for the shareholders. That's the way capitalism works and that's how America became great.

This fact of the manner in which capitalism works, combined with the hunger, fear, and anger cycles created by a carbohydrate diet is what drives the insanity that takes place almost everywhere in the world. It must change if our society is to survive. Monsanto is the driving force behind this corruption and only control of Monsanto will change this. Monsanto needs to own up to their involvement. They need to stop the production of these chemicals that are killing us. They have to stop claiming that their glyphosate is more beneficial than harmful. It isn't and they lie for the benefit of their shareholders, just like most other corporations. We, as consumers, have to stop consuming it. This is the quickest way we can change Monsanto's practices. It may be the quickest way we can save our planet.

I was a very rambunctious kid. I was always getting into some sort of trouble, regardless of what I did. I think is was due to my reluctance to think first, before I acted. This due to my haste in accomplishing my tasks. I was always in a hurry to get my work done. This was due to my lack of patience in seeing the "finished product". I always had trouble finding the patience I needed to competently complete the job my tasks required. Because of this innate inability to constructively accomplish much of what I attempted, i spent a lot of time explaining my motives and actions. This taught not only how to embellish my stories, it taught me that the manner in which I was always trying to do things was completely backwards, due to this innate inability.

Then I discovered that most of this behavior was due to my diet. I just didn't find that out until 4 years ago, 2 years after I quit, eating bread. The trouble I was always in, was usually due to the fact that I couldn't control my emotions. Emotions are always the first to go in a hunger cycle. This is due to the fact that they're controlled by your hormones which are controlled by your diet. This was something that took me 60 years to learn. I wish now that I knew then what I know now, but I couldn't. I was locked into an addiction that kept me from seeing any danger signs except that I needed to make some changes, as that addiction began to wear on me. You see the same changes in yourself, but you didn't know what to do about it, until now.

There is an industry intent on not allowing us to know. That same industry has intentions of using our love of bread for their benefit, seeing an opportunity to make money out of an addiction that we grew into. We've had this affliction all of our lives. We were born into it as it starts before we're born, due to the consumption of it by our mothers who couldn't break away from it. That's because they're born into it. We're all born into it. It's the nature of how this grain has shaped our civilization.

It's shaped our civilization through its hunger cycle which has also forced us to reap the reward of that cycle. Like all cycles, it has its ups and downs and this is what condemns us to the karma we've created through our hunger cycles. When we're hungry, we act with less forethought and concern for long-term consequences of our actions. This doesn't allow us to see all of the possible manifestations of our actions, prior to our committing them. We only see the ones we want to see and this is where we get into trouble. Because of our clouded judgment, we're not open to all possibilities or consequences of those possibilities and this is why our karma comes back to bite us. Too often that karma comes back in the form of terrorism when our hasty decisions are international and affect other people and nationalities. This turns the war on terrorism into a war on hunger and what causes it, sugar and grains, our real nemeses. How many people get angry on a full stomach? Only those with very severe addictions have the power to get mad on a full stomach, as it takes more leptin to satisfy the severely addicted. to evoke the same amount of serotonin.

Due to the fact that this grain has shaped our history so much, it's influenced the overthrow of more territory than any other one reason. Capturing land that grew this important food meant that the conqueror could control the people that this grain fed. That meant security for the owner of such land, provided, he could protect it. It was the wealth that brought this security that drove this kind of behavior, but it was the underlying hunger that drove the desire for security. This is a natural reaction to the hormonal imbalance that the hunger cycle brings with it, everywhere it goes. This is due to the influence that sugar and glucose have on those hormones. They're devastating, to say the least, and they keep your hormones from being under your own control. Because of that, your hormones are under the control of what you're eating. Your diet of carbohydrates makes certain of this.

In my opinion, it's also what leads to all abhorrent behavior that in my eyes is evil. Because this behavior is driven by fear and since fear is what drives all evil, it's my opinion that this food can be considered a driver of evil. It didn't use to be like that, but it is now, especially with the glyphosate that's been dumped, on these crops. Tons of the enzyme inhibiting weed killer is changing our hormonal balance to the point where it's not safe to eat bread anymore. Nor is it safe to eat corn, oats or any grain, for that matter, even sugar. It all gets desiccated before harvest and this is where the danger is, in the desiccating of the crop for a higher yield harvest. This one action alone ensures that we get enough glyphosate into our diets to ensure our compliance with the glucose ruse of a never-ending drug cycle that can only end in a premature death.

All grains (including sugar) are soaked in so much glyphosate that they can't help but rearrange your hormones and ultimately, health. This is why so many people are dying today from all of the modern diseases that exist. This glyphosate actually ramps up the glycation that's responsible for these diseases and disorders, and the general public isn't aware of this. They don't know what's really behind these pandemics of obesity and diabetes, cardiovascular and heart diseases as well as all cancers and dementias. All of this is due to the glycation that this food instigates and the fact that the glycation has been magnified by the glyphosate that it's been drenched in. This is a recipe for disaster for the health of the public. It's a recipe for profit for the pharmaceutical industries. This profit comes from your pockets and your health. Is your addiction worth it?

So, what can you do, to stay away from this glycating sugar in your diet? Nothing, except to give it up...forever. This is the only way you can be free of its addiction, as it's addicted us unwittingly. It did this as soon as we were able to eat it. When one compares the ancient civilizations and their aggressive nature, with the exception of the Huns, the most aggressive civilizations were the ones under the influence of wheat and grains more than anything else. (The Huns benefited from a lack of grain in their diet, making them some of the fiercest warriors. They lived on the milk from the horses.) For the rest of us, these crops became staples in our diet, where they used to only be eaten in small amounts as it took a long time to gather it up, in order to eat it.

The Celtic empire that never had a territory, shows this clearly. The Celts were a tall people. this is due to the protein in the wheat, amylopectin. It enabled the people who ate this einkorn wheat to grow taller and more muscular. What it did underneath the surface was completely hidden until just recently when AGEs were discovered and the real destruction of this kind of diet presented itself. That's in the glycation that these grains create.

The domestication of the grain into crops to feed the masses gave this food, power over the masses and landowners power to control that power. Landowners knew this and that's why they invaded fertile lands first. It was this land that could provide them with enough food to feed their armies. This was the perfect food to feed an army, as you could more easily control this army by controlling their hunger. Powerful warlords knew that whoever controlled the food, controlled the people.

What they didn't know, it was their own hunger that influenced this behavior and that it was the influence of their diets that influenced their hunger. That's something I didn't know until just recently. It took removing them from my diet to fully understand it, but it's plain as day, now that I'm outside of the addiction. One can seldom see an addiction when they're stuck in it and this is the inherent danger in this grain. It's always been addictive, ever since we've been eating it. It always will be and since we've eaten this food all of our lives, we eat it when we're infants, that addicts us unwittingly and forever unless we're aware of its wiles, its dangers, and its addictive allure.

Any substance that affects your hormones like sugar and grains do, is going to be addictive. Alcohol proves this. So does heroin and every other drug. But then so does gambling and all risk-taking, for that fact, because it's driven by a cycle of greed, which is driven by a hunger cycle, which usually pulls, fear, along with it. This is why I contend that all terrorism is driven by a hunger and fear cycle which is driven by sugar and carbs. This is also why I contend that all wars were and are ultimately driven by a hunger and fear cycle because a power grab is a manifestation of a hunger and fear cycle. It's the idea of security that drives someone to gain more power. It's this idea of security that's prompted by the hunger and fear cycle. Hunger and fear, seem to go together. Who wants to go hungry? Because nobody wants to be afraid, they snap into anger to avoid it, automatically. Because I've broken my hunger cycle by breaking my addiction, I can see this clearly, now. It's much easier for you to understand this concept after you break your hunger and fear cycle also. I break it down to this simple equation, grains beget dementia and dementia begets fear. so grains beget fear.

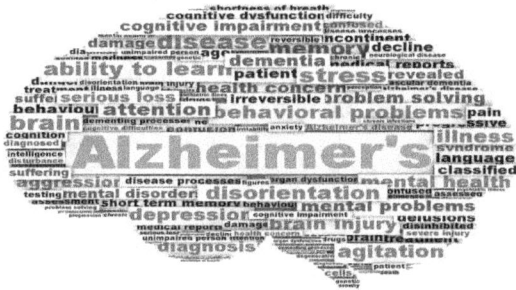

FIND YOUR CURE

THAT YOU KNOW IS PURE

AND LASTS FOREVER THAT'S FOR SURE

BUT, YOU MUST IGNORE THE LURE

TO NOT EAT WHAT IS COMPLETELY IMPURE

WHICH INCLUDES ALL GRAINS, AND THAT'S FOR SURE

VII

THE FDA'S TAKE ON GLUTEN
THE USDA'S CONTROL OF OUR DIET
AND HOW THE INDUSTRY PROFITS

It would be nice if this was a problem with just the grain industry but it's not. It also involves the FDA and what has influenced them to not issue warnings for this allergen and the USDA in recommending what the farm industry can grow the most of. The more I look at it, the more I see that it is a problem with overextending corporate entities. Knowing the dealings that Monsanto has had in the past with competitors and various state and local judicial systems, and in various nations around the world, it's not hard to fathom at all, the involvement they would have, in the cover-up of these studies.

It's actually easy to see their involvement, the same, as that of the sugar industry. The lobbying for their industry is second to none. Remember the name Clarence Thomas, an old Monsanto lawyer and lobbyist, now a Supreme Court Justice. Regulation? According to Monsanto for Monsanto's benefit, alone. Health? That's just collateral damage. Death? That's just collateral damage. Emotional trauma? Again, just collateral damage. Uniting Families? That only happens after it breaks them up.

Gluten does the same thing as sugar. Why can't the FDA recognize that? They have all the studies that point to it. Don't they read them? Why can't they tell us what too much sugar really does? Why can't they tell us about the glycation and the AGEs, and that they lead to all disease? What influences them, not to do so?

The following is an excerpt from an FDA study on Gluten as an allergen (1 of 173 studies).

What is the "Food Allergen Labeling and Consumer Protection Act" (FALCPA) of 2004?

"FALCPA is an amendment to the Federal Food, Drug, and Cosmetic Act and requires that the label of a food that contains an ingredient that is, or contains protein from a "major food allergen " declare the presence of the allergen in the manner described by the law.

Gluten

Why is there a concern about gluten?

"Gluten describes a group of proteins found in certain grains (wheat, barley, and rye.) It is of concern because people with celiac disease cannot tolerate it. Celiac disease (also known as celiac sprue) is a chronic digestive disease that damages the small intestine and interferes with absorption of nutrients from food. Recent findings estimate that 2 million people in the U.S. have celiac disease or about 1 in 133 people".

What does FALCPA require with regard to gluten?

"FALCPA requires FDA to issue a proposed rule that will define and permit the voluntary use of the term "gluten-free" on the labeling of foods by August 2006 and a final rule no later than August 2008". Do they set a safe limit for tar or nicotine in cigarettes? Why do they limit the warning for gluten to a specific amount when it's harmful at any amount?

What has FDA done in *response* to the FALCPA mandate?

"FDA held a public meeting in August 2005 to obtain expert comment and consultation from stakeholders to help FDA develop a regulation to define and permit the voluntary use on food labeling of the term "gluten-free" (Public Meeting On Gluten-Free Food Labeling). The meeting focused on food manufacturing, analytical methods, and consumer issues related to reduced levels of gluten in food." I wonder, did they talk about the glycative effects that get ramped up by the glyphosate? Glycation was actively being studied at the time. Why didn't they discuss that? They had to have known what this food does to the body that consumes it. There are just too many studies showing it.

FDA's gluten-free definition is that the food contains less than 20 ppm of gluten. They actually consider that a warning...of what, I have yet to learn, when the damage is the gluten and should be the warning. Where's the warning, "contains gluten"? Gluten is Latin for glue, you know. Did you ever make paste in grade school? Do you remember what you made it from? My teacher gave me flour and water to make mine. It worked, too, quite well.

What I wonder is, what does the FDA consider stakeholders? Are they the most valuable commodity in this algorithm, the consumers? Or, are they the corporate entities who have an interest in propagating wheat and gluten and the disease, it creates? Since we now know that this happened with sugar, why wouldn't the same thing happen with gluten? We know that gluten breaks down to nothing more than glucose (sugar), I can see where the same situation would exist today, that existed 50-60 years ago. In fact, I believe it's an ongoing problem.

They simply consider wheat and gluten as undeclared allergens yet they refuse to acknowledge its allergenic properties to the extent that they won't require a warning label for it. Yet they know what damage it does. All they require is a mention of wheat in the ingredients and nothing more, and usually, that's in the form of flour. That is their warning. This is tantamount to, only labeling cigarettes that have too much nicotine or tar. Where's the warning about what damage it does, like causing cancer and heart disease, like cigarettes, do? This is actually more of a cause, than cigarettes, for heart disease and cancer. The studies in chapter 4 prove this.

Their negligence in regards to our health in this manner is unconscionable. I can only assume that they've been influenced by the other side of the industry that provides crop seed for the farmers that grow the food that the FDA approves for us to eat. The other side of this industry, owned by the same corporations, is the pharmaceutical industry. They provide us with all of the drugs that we take to fight the pain and disease caused by the food provided by their sister, crop seed/agro-chemical industry.

These are the perpetrators of your Glucose Ruse. They bring to you all of your cases of cancer, CVDs, all dementias, and diseases of inflammation. (If you want someone to thank, you can thank these people, of Monsanto (now, Bayer).

Just like in the tobacco industry, "selling a product that is already sold for them as it's addictive", the same mantra is heard in the grain industry concerning their gluten. "How can people refuse to buy our products? They're addictive so people will want them more. The pizza you love so much is made with high gluten bread dough. That's what damages your stomach and gives you indigestion from eating too much of it. It's not the sauce, spices, toppings or cheese. It's the gluten. It's addictive and that's the taste you crave when you crave pizza. Your indigestion and heartburn is your touch of celiac disease.

I salute the FDA for monitoring products claiming to be gluten-free yet have more than a trace of gluten in them, such as the **Investigation** into General Mills for selling Cheerios that had more than the allowed limit of 20 ppm of gluten. Yet knowing what damage gluten does to the body, I have to wonder why do they still allow it to be marketed without any warnings? The tobacco companies can't market their products without warnings. Why is the food industry allowed to? Don't they ever look at their own studies? The evidence lies within the vaults of the FDA, showing all the damage it does. Why do they ignore that evidence? What evidence, you say? This evidence lies in the excerpts below, from ten of their 173 studies on gluten;

1. *"Gluten is the protein that naturally occurs in wheat, rye, barley, and crossbreeds of these grains. most people can eat gluten, but in people with celiac disease, gluten intake gradually damages the intestines, prevents the absorption of vitamins and minerals, and can lead to other health problems. Symptoms can include diarrhea, fatigue, headaches, abdominal pain, brain fog, rashes, nausea, vomiting, and other reactions."*

2. *"People who have an allergy to wheat run the risk of serious or life-threatening allergic reaction if they eat wheat. Symptoms may include swelling, itching or irritation of mouth or throat, difficulty breathing, nasal congestion, itchy or watery eyes, rash or hives, headaches, nausea, vomiting, cramps, diarrhea, or anaphylaxis, a potentially life-threatening reaction."* What I can't understand; with this kind of disruption of bodily functions, why doesn't this require a warning like cigarettes? It's clearly killed more people.

3. *"unlike food allergies, clinical signs and symptoms do not appear to be reliable markers of disease activity because many individuals affected with celiac disease may be entirely asymptomatic.* This tells me that a lot more people suffer from the disease than what has been diagnosed. *Furthermore, although biomarkers of genetic susceptibility (e.g., presence of dq2 and/or dq8 hla alleles) and gluten exposure [e.g., antibodies for gliadin (aga), endomysial (ema), and tissue transglutaminase (ttg)] have been defined for use in noninvasive diagnosis of individuals with celiac disease, these biomarkers have not been shown to correlate with disease severity nor to be useful in assessing daily responses to gluten exposures. Rather, evidence of intestinal mucosal inflammation is the gold standard biomarker for diagnosis of celiac disease and for assessment of disease severity. Intestinal mucosal inflammation may occur long before the development of clinical signs or a rise in antibody titers following a gluten challenge. Intestinal inflammation is assessed by intestinal biopsy, which is an invasive procedure, associated with false negatives (due to sampling error), and is impractical for frequent monitoring of disease activity or severity."*

4. *"unpublished data described in moneret-vautrin and kanny (2004) show that 83% of wheat allergic children reacted to less than 2 g of wheat flour while only 18% of wheat allergic adults* responded at this level. Unpublished data described in moneret vautrin (2004) on wheat flour *challenges using 32 children and 32 adults with wheat*

allergy, reported a loael of ≤ 1.8 mg protein for allergic children (the lowest tested dose) and 52.8 mg protein for allergic adults. Scibilia et al. (2006) reported that 2 of 13 responders reacted to the lowest dose of wheat flour tested (100 mg of a mix of bread and durum flour, approximately 15 mg protein) in dbpcfcs. In total, 31% of the patients who reacted did so to challenge doses less than or equal to 240 mg of wheat protein." Approaches to establishing thresholds for major food allergens, is what i question, how many people eat this amount? Most people eat around 150mg of wheat products in a day, not enough to express symptoms of celiac disease, but enough to do unnoticed damage. 240 mg/day is almost enough to generate obesity. The fact that it's the instigator of glycation should be enough to warrant a warning similar to what's required for cigarettes.

5. *"the foods of concern for individuals with, or susceptible to, celiac disease are the cereal grains that contain the storage proteins prolamin and glutelin (commonly referred to as gluten in wheat), including all varieties of wheat (e.g., durum, spelt, kamut), barley (where the storage proteins are called hordiens), rye (where the storage proteins are called secalins), and their cross-bred hybrids (such as triticale). The proportion of individuals with celiac disease that are also sensitive to the storage proteins in oats (avenins) has not been determined but is likely to be less than 1% (kelly, 2005)."*

6. *"the clinical manifestations of celiac disease are highly variable in character and severity. The reasons for this diversity are unknown but may depend on the age and immunological status of the individual, the amount, duration, or timing of exposure to gluten, and the specific area and extent of the gastrointestinal tract involved by disease (dewar et al., 2004). These clinical manifestations can be divided into gastrointestinal, or "classic," and non-gastrointestinal manifestations. Gastrointestinal manifestations usually present in children 4 to 24 months old and include abdominal pain and cramping, bloating, recurrent or chronic diarrhea in association with weight loss, poor growth, nutrient deficiency, and (in rare cases) a life-threatening metabolic emergency termed celiac crisis, characterized by hypokalemia and acidosis secondary to profuse diarrhea (farrell and kelly, 2002; baranwal et al., 2003). Non-gastrointestinal manifestations are more insidious and highly variable and are the common presenting signs in older children and adults. These manifestations are frequently the result of long-term nutrient malabsorption, including iron deficiency anemia, short stature, delayed puberty, infertility, and osteoporosis or osteopenia (fasano, 2003). In children, progressive malabsorption of nutrients may lead to growth, developmental, or neurological delays (catassi and fasano, 2004). Extra-intestinal manifestations such as dermatitis herpetiformis, hepatitis, peripheral neuropathy, ataxia, and epilepsy*

have also been associated with celiac disease (fasano and catassi, 2001). Individuals with untreated celiac disease are also at increased risk for potentially serious medical conditions, such as other autoimmune diseases (e.g., type i diabetes mellitus) and intestinal cancers associated with high mortality (farrell and kelly, 2002; peters et al., 2003; catassi et al., 2002). For example, individuals with celiac disease have an 80-fold greater risk of developing adenocarcinoma of the small intestine, a greater than two-fold increased risk for intestinal or extraintestinal lymphomas (green and jabri, 2003) and a 20-fold greater risk of developing enteropathy-associated t cell lymphoma (eatl) (catassi et al.,"

7. "there is no standard protocol for gluten challenges, and challenge studies have varied greatly in amount and duration of gluten exposure. Although some studies have been designed to determine the acute effects (i.e., after 4 hours) of exposure to gluten (sturgess et al., 1994; ciclitira et al., 1984), most challenges consist of an open challenge to a fixed or incremental dose of daily gluten over a minimum period of 4 weeks. Many challenge studies use a high exposure ($\geq$ 10 g/day) to gluten because this is believed to shorten time to disease confirmation or relapse and, therefore, to minimize discomfort to subjects (rolles and mcneish, 1976). However, some studies have shown that low daily exposures to gluten also can elicit a disease response (stassi et al., 1993; laurin et al., 2002; hamilton and mcneill, 1972)."

8. "at this time there is no correlative information on the efficacy of using these tests to predict or help prevent adverse effects in individuals with celiac disease."

9. "although gluten-free diets are considered the only effective treatment for individuals with celiac disease, it has been recognized that it is difficult, if not impossible, to maintain a diet that is completely devoid of gluten (collet al., 2004). Therefore, several attempts have been made to define gluten-free in regulatory contexts. Efforts by the codex alimentarius to define an international standard for "gluten-free" labeling date back to 1981. At that time, due to the lack of sensitive, specific analytical methods, a threshold value of 0.05 g nitrogen per 100 g dry matter was set for wheat starch, on the assumption that wheat protein would be the only source of nitrogen in starch (codex standard 118-1981). The codex committee on nutrition and foods for special dietary uses is developing a revised standard. The current draft proposal would define three categories of gluten-free foods: processed foods that are naturally "gluten-free" ($\leq$ 20 ppm of gluten), products that had been rendered "gluten-free" by processing ($\leq$ 200 ppm), and any mixture of the two ($\leq$ 200 ppm). The australia new zealand food agency (anzfa) defines gluten to mean "the main protein in wheat, rye, oats, barley, triticale and spelt relevant to the medical

conditions, celiac disease, and dermatitis hepetiformis." anzfa recognizes two classes of foods, gluten-free foods (" ...no detectable gluten") and low-gluten foods (" ...no more than 20 mg gluten per 100 gm of the food") (anza food code standard 1.2.8). The canadian standard for "gluten-free" is more general, simply stating that "no person shall label, package, sell or advertise a food in a manner likely to create an impression that it is a "gluten-free" food unless the food does not contain wheat, including spelt and kamut, or oats, barley, rye, triticale or any part thereof" (Canadian food and drugs act regulation b.24.018)." Approaches to establishing thresholds for major food allergens and for gluten in food. Iii, iv, v.
10. *"like food allergies, celiac disease affects only a small proportion of the u.s. population (estimated at 1%, 3.1 million) (nih, 2004). Susceptibility to celiac disease is genetically determined and is linked to the presence of the dq2 or dq8 hla alleles. However, carrying these alleles does not necessarily lead to celiac disease. Both acute and chronic morbidity have been well documented for individuals with symptomatic celiac disease. A gluten-free diet has been shown to greatly reduce the risk for cancer and overall mortality for these individuals. The potential benefit of a gluten-free diet has not been established for individuals with silent or latent celiac disease."*

Now that you know what grains this involves you can get an idea of what not to eat. I submit that this is a disease of a much grander scale, meaning a lot more people suffer from it than what's reported, as far too often this disease goes completely unrecognized (silent) and thus undiagnosed (latent). I hear complaints from many carboholics about many of the disorders at the top of this list. That tells me that they each have an allergic intolerance to gluten and they don't even know it. Because of its addictive nature, they'll never know it, unless they can give it up.

The above paragraphs apply to those with celiac disease, yet I contend that everyone experiences some of the above reactions, to some degree. This happens even more so if you consume more of their products. I thought I could eat this food for 58 years until I learned that I had allergies to it. Now I know that I have allergic intolerances to this food. It presents itself every time I try to eat it again.

My guess is 90% of the population is exactly the same as I am, allergic to the protein in gluten. I contend that the obesity and diabetes rates that exist today confirm this. The death rates of all the diseases caused by gluten prove it. That forces me to ask, with all the evidence available in their archives, why doesn't this food require a warning of the possible diseases it can be the cause of?

What the FDA claims they're concerned about;

"In 21 code of federal regulations (cfr) part 117, we have established our regulation entitled "current good manufacturing practice, hazard analysis, and risk-based preventive controls for human food." We published the final rule establishing part 117 in the federal register of september 17, 2015 (80 fr 55908). Part 117 establishes requirements for current good manufacturing practice for human food (cgmps), for hazard analysis and risk-based preventive controls for human food (pchf), and related requirements."

These codes refer to manufacture and processing of food, but not growing. The FDA, leaves that up to the USDA, which is more concerned for the grower, which is in this case, industrially grown. That is precisely where the danger lies, our food and health, controlled by corporate greed. The FDA cares not, that this poison exists abundantly, in our most heavily eaten foods. They choose to remain ignorant to the fact, endangering your lives. As far as this regulation is concerned, they're failing, in monumental proportions. After reviewing over half of the documents available and an examination of all the titles of the documents, I see nothing that bans the inclusion of any of these dangerous foods in our food products made for public consumption in all processed foods, including bread, pasta and cereal. It seems their interest lies only in compliance with the labeling of the product. They want to make sure that a package that's sold as gluten-free has to have less than 20ppm gluten In the product, meaning, it's OK to eat this poisonous allergen, just not too much of it. I think, Glyphosate has changed their algorithm for calculating the danger this allergen provides and they need to re-assess their thinking and position, on it.

They don't even feel that it's important enough to warn you that a product contains gluten, nor do they feel it important enough to warn you of the dangers of gluten on the package like they do with the dangers of cigarettes. They recognize the danger of tobacco, why can't they recognize the dangers of gluten and wheat? It seems that they're content, with informing you, that a product is gluten-free, even when "gluten-free" doesn't offer any security, but where's the warning, "contains gluten", as if it does no harm at all? "C'MON MAN." I have access to the same studies, they have. They're all located at **PUBMED.COM** and they all explain the dangers this food presents. If I can learn about what this food does, they have to know. Why are they so willing to ignore it? Why are they so willing to treat this food as though there's nothing wrong with it.

The last study on a page of 40 studies, I opened, brought me to this study;

- **"GRAIN AND LEGUME ALLERGY"**

  "Among grains and legumes, wheat and soybean are the most frequent and well-characterized allergenic foods. Wheat proteins are divided into water/salt-soluble and water/salt-insoluble (gluten) fractions. The most dominant allergen in the former is α-amylase/trypsin inhibitor, which acts as an inhaled allergen causing baker's asthma. Gluten allergens, including ω-5 gliadin and high- and low-molecular-weight glutenins, contribute to wheat-dependent exercise-induced anaphylaxis in adults and immediate-type wheat allergies, including anaphylaxis, in children. Recently, wheat allergies exclusively caused by hydrolyzed wheat proteins or deamidated glutens have been reported, and the presence of unique IgE-binding epitopes has been suggested. Soybean allergens contributing to immediate-type allergic reactions in children are present in seed storage proteins, namely Gly m 5, Gly m 6 and Gly m 8. However, pollen-related soybean allergy in adults is caused by the Bet v 1 homolog of soybeans, Gly m 4. Taken together, the varying clinical manifestations of wheat and soybean allergies are predominantly caused by their different allergen components."

In the tenth study on the list published, in July 2009, it's been found that the globulins in wheat can cause type 1 diabetes. T1D is an autoimmune disorder that was thought to have no cause. At least, all the studies I've looked at didn't reveal this.

According to **BioMed Central**;

- **"IDENTIFICATION OF THREE WHEAT GLOBULIN GENES BY SCREENING A TRITICUM AESTIVUM BAC GENOMIC LIBRARY WITH CDNA FROM A DIABETES-ASSOCIATED GLOBULIN"**

  ### Background
  "Exposure to dietary wheat proteins in genetically susceptible individuals has been associated with increased risk for the development of Type 1 diabetes (T1D). Recently, a wheat protein encoded by cDNA WP5212 has been shown to be antigenic in mice, rats and humans with autoimmune T1D. To investigate the genomic origin of the identified wheat protein cDNA, a hexaploid wheat genomic library from Glenlea cultivar was screened."

  ### Results
  Three unique wheat globulin genes, Glo-3A, Glo3-B and Glo-3C, were identified. We describe the genomic structure of these genes and their expression pattern in wheat seeds. The Glo-3A gene shared 99% identity with the cdna of WP5212 at the nucleotide and

deduced amino acid level, indicating that we have identified the gene(s) encoding wheat protein WP5212. Southern analysis revealed the presence of multiple copies of Glo-3-like sequences in all wheat samples, including hexaploid, tetraploid and diploid species wheat seed. Aleurone and embryo tissue specificity of WP5212 gene expression, suggested by promoter region analysis, which demonstrated an absence of endosperm
specific cis elements, was confirmed by immunofluorescence microscopy using anti-WP5212 antibodies.

Conclusion
"Taken together, the results indicate that a diverse group of globulins exists in wheat, some of which could be associated with the pathogenesis of t1d in some susceptible individuals. These data expand our knowledge of specific wheat globulins and will enable further elucidation of their role in wheat biology and human health."

I have read elsewhere that it might be an allergen that triggers an autoimmune response that shuts down the hormones that trigger insulin manufacture in the pancreas. It appears that this is that finding. Wheat can be responsible for type 1 diabetes. Have you seen any warnings for that? I haven't. Have any been issued? I haven't seen them. Why haven't they been issued? How many parents have fed their kids bread to find out that their children are diabetic because of this auto-immune disorder? Why is bread still considered by so many to be a necessity of life? It doesn't appear so. It appears more likely to be a destroyer of life.

What I'm concerned about;
47,397 deaths daily from CVDs

47,397 people died each day, worldwide, from cardiovascular disease in 2013. That breaks down to over 1800 americans that died every day from cardiovascular disease in 2013. That's 17.3 million annually, worldwide. That was up from 12.3 million (25.8%) in 1990. According to **Wikipedia**;

"coronary artery disease and stroke account for 80% of cvd deaths in males and 75% of cvd deaths in females, the most cardiovascular disease affects older adults. In the united states, 11% of people between 20 and 40 have cvd, while 37% between 40 and 60, 71% of people between 60 and 80, and 85% of people over 80 have cvd. The average age of death from coronary artery disease in the developed world is around 80 while it is around 68 in the developing world." This rate is increasing each year right alongside the use of glyphosate.

This points to the fact that this food which is eaten on a daily basis does so little damage incrementally to the consumer that it's never noticed until it's too late. The disease has already manifested itself and the price is now being paid for a lifetime of consumption. The question I keep asking myself is why does this have to keep happening? Why hasn't the FDA warned us about the dangers of this food? They have access to all of the same reports that I do, yet they still refuse to acknowledge that this food is dangerous. Does their interest lie elsewhere? I'm forced to wonder, is there **corporate influence** involved with this like there was with sugar?

ACCORDING TO THE GUARDIAN;

- ***"SUGAR LOBBY PAID SCIENTISTS TO BLUR SUGAR'S ROLE IN HEART DISEASE REPORT"***

    "New report highlights battle by the industry to counter sugar's negative health effects, and the cushy relationship between food companies and researchers Influential research that downplayed the role of sugar in heart disease in the 1960s was paid for by the sugar industry, according to a report released on monday. "the sugar industry actively took steps for years to influence public's perception of the nutritional value of their product, when they clearly knew of the dangers it posed. "food companies have spent billions of dollars to cover up the link between sugar consumption and health problems. That's the conclusion of a new **report** *from the center for science and democracy at the union of concerned scientists (ucs)."*

These actions are responsible for more deaths than all the world wars combined. Their actions have killed, hurt or harmed more than 900,000,000 people in the last 30 years alone. (At 17.3 million/yr for heart disease alone, 900 million is a lowball estimate for death coming from cancer and dementia as well.) All total, the death rate for **ECC** is over 30,000,000 each year. That's over 82,191 deaths each day, simply from excessive carbohydrate consumption.

"With backing from a sugar lobby, scientists promoted dietary fat as the cause of coronary heart disease instead of sugar", according to a historical document review published in JAMA Internal Medicine. This was criminal, yet nothing was done about it.

Though the review is nearly 50 years old, it also showcases a decades-long battle by the sugar industry to counter the product's negative health effects. Why isn't this agency being held accountable?

The findings come from documents recently found by a researcher at the University of San Francisco, which show that scientists at the Sugar Research Foundation (SRF), known today as the sugar association, paid scientists to do a 1967 literature review that overlooked the role of sugar in heart disease. I would consider this criminal intent that should have been investigated, wouldn't you?

> *"SRF set an objective for the review, funded it and reviewed drafts before it was published in the new england journal of medicine, which did not require conflict of interest disclosure until 1984. The three harvard scientists who wrote the review made what would be $50,000 in today's dollars from the review".*

Because of this criminality, close to 1billion have suffered, immensely, from these diseases that sugar is responsible for, in the last 30 years alone. From diabetes to heart disease to arthritis to cancer to...you should know the list by now. They've been spraying this herbicide for more than 40 years, making 1 billion victims, a very lowball estimate.

> *Marion nestle, a nutrition, food studies and public health professor at New York University, said* ***"the food industry continues to influence nutrition science,"*** *in an editorial published alongside the JAMA report.*

When will it stop? Never, until we let this industry know that we won't accept their definition of healthy food and stop buying their versions of it. That, is the only control we have over this pitfall, indulge, or resist the addiction. That's our choices, thanks to Monsanto.

> *"Today, it is almost impossible to keep up with the range of food companies sponsoring research – from makers of the most highly processed foods, drinks, and supplements to producers of dairy foods, meats, fruits, and nuts – typically yielding results favorable to the sponsor's interests," nestle said. "food company sponsorship, whether or not intentionally manipulative, undermines public trust in nutrition science, contributes to public confusion about what to eat, and compromises dietary guidelines in ways that are not in the best interest of public health."*
>
> *"The cushy relationship between food companies and researcher has been captured in recent investigations by the*

associated press and New York Times." The AP revealed in June that candy trade groups were funding research into sweets. And in 2015, the new york times showed how coca-cola has funded millions in research to downplay the link between sugary beverages and obesity.

The sugar association said in a statement, "SRF should have exercised greater transparency" in its research, but also accused the study authors of having an "anti-sugar narrative".

"we question this author's continued attempts to reframe historical occurrences to conveniently align with the currently trending anti-sugar narrative, particularly when the last several decades of research have concluded that sugar does not have a unique role in heart disease," the sugar association said. "most concerning is the growing use of headline-baiting articles to trump quality scientific research – we're disappointed to see a journal of jama's stature being drawn into this trend."

"The findings were based on documents found by kristin kearns, a postdoctoral fellow at ucsf, in library archives. The scientists and executives involved are no longer alive."

"In recent years, the link between fat and heart disease has become a more contentious topic – a 2010 review of scientific studies of fat in the American Journal of Clinical Nutrition found that there is no convincing evidence that saturated fat causes heart disease. The role of sugar in heart disease is still being debated."

Even according to **Mother Jones**; *"the industry's tactics—similar to those used by big tobacco in downplaying the adverse health effects of smoking—were explored by Gary Taubes and Cristin Kearns Couzens in the 2012 Mother Jones investigation* **"Big Sugar's Sweet Little Lies**.*" but this latest report draws on some* **newly released documents** *submitted as evidence in a recent federal court case involving the two biggest players in the sweetener industry: the sugar association and the corn refiners association (the trade group for manufacturers of high fructose corn syrup)."*

The evidence is piling up!
The FDA can't hide their complicity much longer.

"Obesity and diabetes mellitus are often linked to cardiovascular disease, as are a history of chronic kidney disease and hypercholesterolemia.In fact, cardiovascular disease is the most life-threatening of the diabetic complications and diabetics are two- to four-fold more likely to die of cardiovascular-related causes than nondiabetics."

> "Up to 90% of cardiovascular disease may be preventable if established risk factors are avoided. "their goal is 25 by 25". 25x25 is a goal of achieving a 25% relative reduction in overall mortality from cardiovascular disease, cancer, diabetes or chronic respiratory disease by 2025. In september 2011, the united nations held a high-level meeting in new york on the subject of ncds, including cardiovascular disease (cvd), cancers, diabetes and chronic respiratory diseases."

They're actively taking steps to lower the death rate of CVDs by recommending everyone to eat right, quit smoking, and exercise, all of which will lower this number one killer of people. Eating right, in my opinion, is by far the best way to combat CVDs, diabetes, obesity, hypertension, high cholesterol (which is really a problem of unbalanced cholesterol), arthritis and worst of all, dementia and Alzheimer disease.

In all of my research, I can't find anything that says to limit the use of bread and starchy carbohydrates made from grains, (with the exception of a growing number of doctors who endorse the ketogenic diet). Yet all research I've looked at from PubMed and even the FDA show that this food does cause these disorders. Every time I look at the data, I'm forced to ask myself, why hasn't' the FDA, WHA, (World Health Administration) or the ADA condemned this food? These agencies have to know what's going on, yet they refuse to act. Who is blocking this action?

After researching my book *IT'S TIME FOR A CURE*, I've learned that this food is at the base of **all** major disease, forcing me to ask, why hasn't the FDA or the WHF (World Heart Federation) warned us of this food. The only reason I can come up with is that it is being protected from prosecution by the industry that provides the crop seed for the farmer as well as the chemicals for the drugs to combat the arthritis caused by what their seed grows into.

From PubMed's study;
- **Characterization of Proteins from Grain of Different Bread and Durum Wheat Genotypes:**
"wheat is unique among the edible grains because wheat flour has the protein complex called "gluten" that can be formed into the dough with the rheological properties required for the production of leavened bread. The rheological properties of gluten are needed not only for bread production but also in the wider range of foods that can only be made from wheat, viz., noodles, pasta, pocket bread, pastries, cookies, and other products. The gluten proteins

consist of monomeric gliadins and polymeric glutenins. Glutenins and gliadins are recognized as the major wheat storage proteins, constituting about 75–85% of the total grain proteins with a ratio of about 1:1 in common or bread wheat and they tend to be rich in asparagine, glutamine, arginine or proline but very low in nutritionally important amino acids lysine, tryptophan and methionine"

"Very low in nutritionally important amino acids" interests me. Amino acids are proteins and these proteins are cell signaling proteins, meaning they influence your hormones. This is the ultimate effect of the glyphosate poisoning. If you take away the protein, what do you have left? Carbohydrates, and they're the deadly kind, glyphosated.

This fact combined with the fact that gliadins have been shown to provoke the body to release anti-gliadin antibodies, which also have been shown to have the ability to attach themselves to Purkinje cells in the cerebellum, make this food suspect, at the least. When an anti-gliadin antibody attaches itself to a Purkinje cell in the cerebellum, the brain renders that cell useless and discards it. Although many parts of your brain can grow new cells to replace discarded cells, this area of the brain, can't. That means whenever an anti-gliadin antibody attaches itself to a Purkinje cell, that part of the brain never comes back. Yes, that does mean brain damage for those who release these anti-gliadin antibodies. Do you know if you do?

How many of us release these antibodies? Judging from the amount of Alzheimer's disease invading the civilized world, I would say a majority of people display this form of intolerance....a rather large majority. The next question this conjures is, am I one of them? Are you one of them? I found out that I am. Have you yet?

42,657 deaths worldwide from cardiovascular disease

Heart disease kills more people every year than any other single cause. Over 42,000 people die from this disease each and every day and the only reason it exists is the high amount of sugar we put into our bodies. It brings about the glycation **ECC** is responsible for and it's this glycation that is responsible for at least 42,000 deaths from cardiovascular disease, alone, every day.

But that's not all it is responsible for. We have to look at Alzheimer's disease and dementia. We have to consider cancer, and we have to worry about the amount of high blood pressure and high cholesterol ECC is responsible for. All of these disorders are money producing diseases that this industry generates, simply for the sake of profit. It's this drive for profit that is killing everyone, again showing the lack of responsibility of capitalism.

13,698 deaths globally from Alzheimer disease

13,698 die each day, worldwide, due to Alzheimer disease alone. That amounts to over 500 deaths daily in the US alone, which means that at least 20 people in this country will die this hour, due to Alzheimer disease. Nothing contributes to Alzheimer disease as much as bread consumption. It's the starchy carbs that break down to glucose, and it's the glucose that glycates the cholesterol and protein that builds up the plaque and inflammation in your blood that leads to Alzheimer disease, cancer, arthritis, Atherosclerosis as well as most all other CVDs, as well as hypertension and high cholesterol. The saddest part of this story, it's completely correctable, yet we didn't have any clue as to how to correct it until recently. Thanks to a few good doctors with Perlmutter leading the charge..

11,232 deaths daily from cancer worldwide

11,232 people die every day globally due to some form of cancer and with all the evidence available that wheat contributes to the spread of multiple forms of cancer, why hasn't the FDA made any statements about the dangers this food presents to the human body? Evidence shows these devastating effects going back to the bones of earliest cavemen that have been discovered.

I recently watched a Nova program on a 5,000-year-old ice mummy that had been frozen in a receding ice flow until he was discovered in 1991. They found remnants of einkorn wheat in his upper digestive tract suggesting his last meal was bread made from the flour of einkorn wheat. His bones also showed "disease of a modern lifestyle", as they like to call it. What is this disease of a modern lifestyle? Arthritis. This is evidence of the glycation that occurred in this man from eating the carb-loaded bread made from einkorn wheat. Even as difficult as it was to digest einkorn wheat at that time, due to its fibrous nature, it still did the same damage then, that it does today to everyone who continues to eat this food, today.

IT'S A SIMPLE DECISION TO FORESTALL YOUR PAIN

ALL YOU HAVE TO DO IS GIVE UP THE GRAIN

VIII

USDA'S ABILITY TO MASK THE TAINTING OF THE GRAIN SO THE "FARMER CAN SELL MORE" (TO ADD TO YOUR PAIN)

These industries and agencies are directly responsible for well over 30,000,000 deaths each and every year. That toll continues to climb and it will continue until everyone decides that it's time for a cure.

Decisions have been made in the past that clearly benefited industry while presenting clear dangers to humans. By, not only allowing contaminated food with worthless nutritional values or food contaminated by bacteria to sneak into our food supply, but by polluting our rivers and lakes in the process as well, with contaminated groundwater from runoff with chemical fertilizers, pesticides, and herbicides. All of this is doing undue damage to bee populations, monarch populations, and our whole ecosystem by tainting all of our air and groundwater as well as foliage that these species feed on.

This is just a taste of how unsustainable this is and it all starts with the grain industry, and our insatiable appetites for high sugar food, which is all forced upon up by this industry, the soy and corn producers, wheat growers, and the crop seed companies owned by Monsanto, Syngenta, Bayer, **et al**. Because this food requires treatment with medications that this industry controls, they have full control over what happens inside your body when you bend to their will and buy their products.

The Iowa Corn Fed Beef Ruse

The grain industry in Iowa promoted *Iowa corn-fed beef*, to sell more corn, their largest industry. This had multiple, unforeseen consequences that not only damaged our food supply, but it polluted our resources more than what could have ever been foreseen, by dumping tons of glyphosate into our environment and diets. As instructed by the chemical industry, they dumped tons of glyphosate in the environment to increase their production. This had many unforeseen consequences, tainting bee and monarch habitats, as well as tainting ground water with their chemicals.

Because of our propensity to feed our addiction to sugar, the products that this industry has devised to get us to eat more of their junk food, are putting everyone who is suckered into this cycle, in the hospital with serious disorders. These disorders range from arthritis to cancer to HBP to CVDs and much more, but then, you know by now, what they are.

This is a clear indication of where, self-regulating, doesn't work. It's killing Americans right now because it doesn't. Evidence can be seen in the number of heart disease deaths, cancer deaths, Alzheimer's deaths, not to mention all the pain, discomfort, and drug abuse caused by the pain. Although this is nice for the profits Monsanto, Syngenta and Bayer who also make drugs that treat the diseases their foods cause, it's leading our country down a path of destruction that we'll never recover from if we keep eating the food they advertise. They are playing this addiction, that they keep worsening, on the American people as well as the world to pad their profits and boost their influence. I don't know about you, but I don't like being played like a card or rolled like dice, for someone else's benefit.

This industry makes sure that sugar gets into baby food, to make sure that every baby who eats it becomes addicted to it, making them lifetime users of their poison. This forced addiction to sugar has brought this industry to a level of evil that's never been seen in any industry. This industry is so intent on keeping us addicted to its lure, simply to increase their profits, that they are now responsible for over 82,191 deaths, worldwide, daily. Yes, I said 82,191 deaths daily. If this doesn't bother you, then you have no conscience. Yes, this is something to be appalled about and appalled I am and you should be too. This is simply more proof that it's time for a cure.

From 50,000 food safety inspections in 1972 to barely over 9,000 in 2008, the FDA is failing us on an unprecedented scale. If inspections decreased this much in 36 years, how much do think they've decreased in 46 years? This is directly related to departmental cutbacks reducing the number of agents available to do the inspections.

This is how conservative politicians think this industry and all other industries should regulate themselves. It would be nice if corporate America was concerned about more than just their profits, but unfortunately, the bottom line is what wins, here, and the bottom line is the greed of how, corporate bylaws, require corporations to bend, regulatory law, to increase their profits for shareholders.

If the FDA can allow foods this dangerous through its monitoring, I'm afraid to even think about what else has snuck through? The beef industry has already displayed their contempt for regulation through the mass production of contaminated beef that their industry has been responsible for, in the last 50 years.

We now know for sure that wheat can kill? What I would rather ask, what outside influence was there, in their decision to not issue any warnings? It was recently revealed that the sugar industry took steps to cover up the reports of damage that their food offered, so why wouldn't it make sense that this closely related industry, the grain industry, would take those same steps to cover up the same information about what their foods provide?

Was this another case of the industry regulating itself and its watchdog, as well? Does this make a solid argument, for self-regulation for corporate entities, instead of government regulations? Our health is at stake here and we've allowed the FDA to escape judgment. That in my estimation is borderline criminal. 3,287 deaths nationally, each day from CVDs, cancer, and Alzheimer disease combined. All three of these disorders are directly due to ECC, excessive carbohydrate consumption, which can be controlled. That's enough people to wipe out 4 towns, the same size I grew up in. That's unconscionable and we let it happen. Wouldn't you say, "that is a shame on us", for allowing it to happen?

We have direct control of these disorders. We don't have to let this continue, but we do, simply to feed our addiction. We have a societal addiction to glucose because it's not just sugar, it's what breaks down to glucose, and that includes not only sugar but all carbohydrates that break down to their most basic molecule, glucose. It's our addiction to this glucose that clouds our judgment, masks our emotions, and controls our desires by gumming up the neurons in our brains every time we eat this food. This is exactly what makes it addictive and hands total control over to the glucose, every time we eat it.

Yes, we do have full control over this, and we can stop it, but we have to stop the celebration of our addiction, to stop the addiction itself. To do that we need to be educating the public on the damage it's doing when you eat this food. It's time to show where this hits abusers, in the pocketbook, where it hurts the most.

A tobacco tax has been somewhat successful with cigarettes, in curbing consumption. Eventually, a glucose tax may become law, but if we as consumers, act responsibly now and stop consuming this poisonous food, laws and regulations won't have to control it. We will. That may be our only chance to break this cycle of addiction and destruction because, right now, all laws and regulation are under the control of Monsanto and it's in their benefit to keep this, "status quo".

MONSANTO, THE USDA AND THE FDA

The FDA'S & USDA'S control is the equivalency of Monsanto's control (now, Bayer's). Just like in the tobacco industry, "selling a product that is already sold as it's addictive", the same mantra is heard in the grain industry concerning their gluten. This industry has it easier, your addiction is built-in and doesn't have to be started, like that of cigarettes. *"How can people refuse to buy our products? They're addictive so people will want them more. Better yet, they're legal to sell to kids, "once we hook them, we've got them for life."* So, they do.

I salute the FDA for monitoring products claiming to be gluten-free yet have more than a trace of gluten in them, such as the Investigation into General Mills for selling Cheerios that had more than the allowed limit of 20 ppm of gluten. Yet knowing what damage gluten does to the body, I have to wonder why do they still allow it to be marketed without any warnings of the damage it does? The tobacco companies can't market their products without warnings. Why is the food industry allowed to?

The evidence, against its safety, lies within the databases of the FDA, showing all the damage it does, through its glycative nature. Why do they ignore that evidence and the fact that all grains, sugar, and vegetables get glyphosated? Or are they controlled by outside influences that stand to lose the bulk of their business, if this information were to ever leak out?

Let's look at their shirk of responsibility, a corporation or industry of corporations would stand to lose millions of dollars if this Information were to ever leak out. What corporation would stand to lose the most if this information was known by the public at large, as common knowledge? What corporation(s) has more dollars tied up in this ruse than any other corporation(s)?

To understand that, we need to look at which corporations benefit most from today's cycle of dependence on sugar. It's this cycle of dependence that drives all advertising for all the foods that do the most damage, food like bread, sugary drinks, and snacks made from grains, not necessarily in that order. I put bread first, simply because of its prevalence of being eaten in every meal, every snack and every lunch bucket. Bread starts glycating as soon as it hits your mouth. The plaque on your teeth is proof.

Plaque is a product of glycation. This is similar to the plaque that builds up in your arteries causing most cardiovascular diseases as well as high blood pressure. I know, I was there with high blood pressure. I still have high blood pressure, but I control mine with my diet and nothing else. Right now my blood pressure is 94/63 and my pulse is at 80. I don't take any medication for my HBP. I say that not only to brag (it's one of the few things I have to brag about), but mostly to let you know that you too can do the same as I have done. It's rather simple. Not always easy, but simple. I won't eat grains, root vegetables, fruit or anything that has any sugar in it.

Since I've learned what sugar does, I quit putting that substance in my body. It just brings too many disorders with it. That's the difference in my diet and yours that keeps your blood pressure high enough to keep you on medication. If your high blood pressure is coupled with diabetes, your days are already numbered unless you take immediate action to give up the bread and grains. Anyone who says otherwise is fighting the addiction themselves, and can't see the real truth.

The real truth is, your body doesn't need to digest carbohydrates to survive because carbs are sugar and sugar glycates. Glycation is deadly. You know that by now. It's multiplied when the carbs have little or no fiber, which all grains (cereal and legumes) have. You should know by now, how many disorders it's responsible for initiating. And by that, you should know how many disorders would not exist if you took the glycating sugar away. If you get hungry often, the worse off you are. If you get hungry at all, you're displaying signs of your dependence on sugar. You do this as your blood sugar levels rise and fall according to the number of carbs you put in your mouth. This gives control of your body over to the food that influences this cycle the most, and that's your carbohydrate diet. So the question to ask yourself is, where is your carb diet coming from? Who influences you to buy the bread, corn chips, snack crackers, and soda that promotes this glycation? Aunt Jemima? Uncle Ben? Nabisco? Frito-Lay? Pepsi or Coca-Cola? Or is it every major food vendor in the industry?

INDUSTRY'S ENJOYMENT AT YOUR EXPENSE

It would be nice if money weren't the primary motivating factor in business. It would be nice if the health and welfare of every individual human being was the primary motivating factor in business.

But it's not. It may never be, unless people learn to take account for their addictions and change this behavior that's imbedded in our society. That could well be, never, or until they all die and stop perpetuating the ruse.

That is why this section may be the hardest one to construct. It not only involves corporate America, it involves a major portion of all industry. both big and small, Even down to the mom and pop stores in small town, America, and that's what makes this so hard to confront.

The problem is that this problem invades the very core of our society, our sustenance. This is what we all work for. Our primary goal for our families, (after finding shelter) is to put food on the table. And this is where the problem begins. Everyone has to eat. This makes everyone, who's hungry, susceptible to outside influences, to quell those hunger pangs.

The food industry understands this. They've done numerous studies on it. Their research has told them how, when, where, and to whom to market their products. All so they can increase their profits. Their only interest, is to please their stockholders, they're not interested in their customer's health (unless they're in the health industry), so everything they do, is done for the bottom line, profit. I'm beginning to think that this is Monsanto's version of population control. It's cutting short the lives of over 52,000 people, every day. Can you imagine a city the size of Casper, WY disappearing every day? We live with that equivalency.

These products kill because of the sugar they contain, we all know that. But the problem, here is, that they don't kill immediately. Their death sentence takes a lot longer. It's a lot more painful. It's a lot more expensive. It's a lot more emotionally draining. It's definitely, nothing anyone should have to experience, yet the addiction keeps anyone who's on this diet, remain on this diet, voluntarily. Only those strong enough can break the cycle of addiction. But the beauty of breaking it is this, it doesn't take that long, as long as you can abstain from its lure. It only takes a month or two, for the average addict. Heavier, more addicted people, might take another month or two. But I can promise you, that everyone will experience the magic of partial freedom, even by abstaining for the period of time, they can. They just have to give it an honest attempt, longer than 2 weeks. The easiest way to start is a 3 day water-only fast, and when you start eating again, eat no carbs.

Bringing the food industry to an understanding, that they are sacrificing tomorrow's customers for today's profits, may help in curbing corporate influence, but is it enough to change the behavior of all corporate America? I don't know. The amount of change that would have to occur, is enormous because the industry is enormous. How do you change an industry this enormous? The only way I know how to is by removing the need for their product, which unfortunately, can only be done by breaking an addiction.

Unfortunately, profit doesn't have a soul. It has no moral values. And it's the moral values that make us a society. Without them, we'd have no laws or regulations to keep people from hurting each other. This begs the question, what role does profit play in a civilized culture. Most of us know that profit = money. Most of us also know that a civilization needs money to conduct commerce, so everyone within that civilization can trade their goods and services. It's this trade, that's at the core of civilization. People came together during the stone age mostly to grow grain crops we used to forage on. Because this provided year around food, it in turn, started us trading our possessions and food. This was basically the start of agriculture. And thus, the beginning of commerce, the engine that keeps our society, culture, and civilization growing.

If it's the desire of money, that's at the root of all evil, does that make all of corporate America evil, because of their desire to improve their profits? Some would say so, simply due to the lack of responsibility, corporate America takes for their actions when they harm others. Others would say, it's survival. In all actuality, it's both. The desire for profit and power is what drives almost all of corporate America. In my opinion, this is where corporate America is failing society.

Because they have to fulfill stockholders wishes to make more money, they are obligated to do so. Doing anything else would not be considered profitable and it wouldn't keep the stockholders happy. The company would lose the investment of their stockholders and this, in turn, would strongly disable their ability to conduct business and therein threaten the existence of the company. Profit is important. It's one of the biggest, if not the biggest motivating factors in our society.

We, in the United States, have always used our freedoms, to bolster our efforts to increase our profits. It's this freedom, that's built the strongest empire in history. The problem is this when you consider freedom and what it brings us, you have to look at the other side of the coin, that freedom is on. The other side of this freedom coin, that's tossed around so much (mostly politically), is responsibility. You can't have true freedom without responsibility. The responsibility side of the coin, says, that you must take responsibility for the freedoms you enjoy, especially when those freedoms inflict harm on another human being. You can't have true freedom without this responsibility. Without the responsibility, what do you have? A society without control. When anybody, person, group, or company isn't fully responsible for enjoying their freedoms, where does the freedom exist for all parties? Isn't that called slavery?

It's how our system, works, and because our Supreme Court thinks that corporations are the same as people, they've said that they deserve the same rights and freedoms as any single individual human being. Yet, they're allowed a lot more freedom, simply because, they have the money to do so. Here's the worst part of this algorithm, because of our addiction, it's our money they use. We give it to them, freely, every time we buy their products. What we think we do on our own, is really the drive of the glucose change in our hormones, which is in their control. We're actually succumbing to their desire. You are slaves to their wishes, when you eat their glyphosated foods.

This is a trap, that I refuse to fall into. I can only thank Dr Perlmutter, Dr Davis, and Dr Amen, for setting me on the path that brought me to this point, and all these books, (I don't mention Dr. Amen anywhere, except right here. The reason I mention him here, is because he's the one who basically started me on this journey.)

Why does this ruse, continue? In one word, profit. Shareholders demand it. corporate bylaws demand it. By law, many of them have to take part in this ruse, just to pay dividends. Consumers demand it, to feed their addiction. This is the inherent problem with corporate capitalism. What moves America forward, more than anything else is a corporate advancement. Hence the control of corporations in America is what controls this advancement but it's profit that drives it.

If any major change is to occur within the realms of modern society, it must be done, by diminishing, demand for this substance. This brings us to the dilemma of how to change the behavior of millions of people, all who are addicted to these substances and worse yet addicted to what corporate America tells them. They tell them how to think, how to eat, what to drink, primarily what they should be eating and drinking. This puts them in control of the amount of sugar we consume, which in turn, controls our emotions, to put us 'under their spell', so to speak. They're never going to want to give that up. That's something that we have to take back. In order to effect, changes in the food industry, primarily the grain industry, we need to make corporate America know, that we're tired of their abuse.

It must be incorporated into this network of our society, that change must happen. The problem therein lies, this industry is huge. It's comprised of, probably more companies, than any other industry, in the world, as food is the most important commodity that's marketed worldwide. The number of companies within this industry is almost unimaginable. So how do we change the behavior of this much of our society? It can't be done overnight. It's going to take the efforts of everyone in society, to make a change, this grandiose, which means it's going to take a while. That's why we need to start yesterday.

Corporate industry, the food industry primarily, must confront the dangers, that they are imposing on the entire world, by continuing to grow, manufacture, market, advertise and sell this devastating food that causes so many illnesses and diseases. They must understand that killing their customers, is not a solid business plan, that is, if you want to keep your customer base. Unless, they think that cycling a never-ending line of clients, all waiting to be inflicted, blindly, is more profitable. It's too bad, they can't put humanity, first.

I realize that many of the crop seed companies, (Monsanto, DuPont, Syngenta, Land O' Lakes, Bayer and many others overseas), have a lot of the money tied up in pharmaceuticals, as well as manufacturing the crop seed, (much of it genetically modified). Even though many of those companies liquidated their investments in the pharmaceutical side of the industry, many of these companies still have ties to each other, which begs the question, were cover-ups initiated to help hide these facts? It conjures, in my mind, the question of how threatened did they feel if any of this information was released to the public?

With corporate America in so much control of how our society functions, it's occurred to me that nothing is going to happen, until corporate America, the food industry and pharmaceutical industry, in general, change their behavior, They must discontinue the marketing and advertising of these products, so as to not persuade the public that they need to continue to eat this garbage. The question arises, how do you make a company cut its own throat. Because if anything were to interrupt the flow of their finances, how long can they stay in business? This brings us to the core of what we need to work toward to change, and changing it, may result in much of this industry transitioning to other industries and markets.

The drink industry, for example, they're probably the guiltiest of any, for slipping this dangerous food into our diet, by loading up their drinks with **high-fructose corn syrup, sugar, Aspartame, Cyclamate, Saccharin, Sucralose, Acesulfame potassium, malt syrup, Lead acetate**, and many others that I have trouble pronouncing, like **maltodextrin, maltitol, maltotriose, Icodextrin**, and too many forms of **oligosaccharides** to list here. To find them all, you need to refer to every food label on every can of soft drink, that's on the market. Convincing the beverage industry of finding other sources of sweeteners is already beginning to take place. A lot of manufacturers are starting to offer drinks sweetened with stevia, a completely natural, non-caloric sweetener, that's super concentrated when it's offered in powdered form. My wish is for the transformation of all sweetened drinks to stevia or glycerol, instead of the high sugar sweeteners, like of those listed above. I know of some people who use glycerol, as it's a natural sweetener that is a lipid, meaning it comes without the glycating effects that sugar comes with. Can you imagine what this would do, to get this dangerous substance, glucose, out of our diet? I'm just beginning to.

So how do we replace the lost business and everything else that goes along with it, the jobs and careers, the investment of millions of Americans, who've all invested in these companies(through their IRA'S, Keoghs, investment funds, etc)? How do we take away all of that? The problem is, you can't, and that's where the problem of dispelling this problem, lies. You have to replace what you take away, with healthier options, healthier for the body, healthier for business and corporate America. My contention is that business or corporate America, and the health of the individual run hand in hand. They depend on each other. They're crucial to each other's survival. The problem with this equation, is that corporate America uses this against us, forcing us to need their medications. They actually think that making us ill is a good business model for them, as it forces our need for their medicine. I call this unsustainable.

Why then, doesn't the food industry understand this basic fundamental law of business, that killing your customers with inferior products, is killing your industry? Unless that industry is still working with the pharmaceutical industry like they were 30 - 40 years ago. Could they be that indebted to the pharmaceutical industry, that they have to keep sending them customers?

I mentioned before that Monsanto is now controlled by Bayer. Last year Bayer and Monsanto merged, and with Bayer being the larger of the two corporations, they now control Monsanto and your food supply. If I still ate these foods, I'd be concerned. I definitely wouldn't be comfortable eating what an Eastern European pharmaceutical company is giving me to eat. Next year, that's going to be the case for all those, not on a ketogenic diet. I pity them. This is probably the only warning you'll ever get.

THE PRICE TO PAY FOR GOOD HEALTH.

There is a price to pay for good health, and you can pay it while you eat and years later with medications, or you can buy your good health with what you eat. It does matter what you decide to put in your mouth if you're going to keep your body healthy or not. You can pay now, with good food or you can pay later in medical costs. (Even insurance won't be able to help curb your costs enough in the future.)

Of all the good things that have happened to me, this is undoubtedly the most beneficial one of them. My mind is now clearer and better at reasoning than it's been in the last 33 years since I suffered the severe closed head injury that I live with. For thirty years my recovery was basically static. That was until I learned what's behind inflammation and all modern diseases.

We've been urged to believe that the guilty party in our blood is our cholesterol when in all reality it's the glucose or sugar that we continuously want to feed our bodies. And, an industry with massive amounts of money tied up in grains and sugar, has purposely impressed their idea of healthy food on us, much to our dismay, as it's what they're promoting that's making everyone die prematurely from cancer, heart diseases like atherosclerosis, inflammatory heart disease, and all brain disorders such as Alzheimer's disease, Parkinson's disease. dementia of any type due to the destructive action of the glucose on your cholesterol and protein cells.

That means that the only really healthy diet to be on is a ketogenic diet. Mine is an MCT keto diet due to the balancing of cholesterol that it provides. The ultimate in good health is only found with high cholesterol levels. That's because your body uses cholesterol more than the grain industry wants you to know.

They're doing their best to vilify cholesterol, yet it's the glucose that creates the glycation and it's the glycation that is at the root of all modern disease and physical and mental disorder. Doesn't that make glucose the real villain in this tale of woe? This is the heart of your Glucose Ruse.

Since the body loves fat, I feed mine fat. It seems to love it too. Without the glucose in my system, I have no glycation in my blood to create any inflammation, pain, disease, mental or physical disorder of any sort. This gives my body a better ability to fight off every other disease, whether bacterial or viral. In other words, I don't get sick. I don't get headaches. I don't get stomach aches. I don't get colds. I don't get the flu. The only problem I have is my allergies, unfortunately, I've shown to be allergic to 72 out of 88 allergens when last tested. But then, that was prior to my change in diet. More important than the lack of inflammation in my body is the lack of inflammation in my brain, and that's exactly what drags down, every other brain on a grain diet down. It's the inflammation that the glycation creates in the body. It also creates it in the brain.

The lack of inflammation in my brain over the last 5 years has allowed me to compile 16 paperbacks and ebooks, 10 of those in the last year alone. All of this while maintaining 8 websites. My abilities to accomplish this is simply due to my change in diet to no carbs and more fat and protein to give my brain what it needs to grow smarter every day. Quite possibly, the best benefit I've gotten out of this change is the lack of need for me to take any medication. Even though I still have to deal with break-through pain, I take absolutely no pills for it. What I use now is completely natural and has no ill effects on my body or brain.

I can remember many times in my youth when I was a toddler, a steady stream of snot running from my nose to my mouth, most of the time. Whenever Mom saw it, she always said, "Chip, cut that out. When your nose runs like that, wipe it off with a Kleenex and blow your nose, that's disgusting". It probably appeared disgusting, but for me, I was recycling. I was just putting back to use that which was vacating my sinuses.

What's unfortunate is that my mom didn't know what it was that was making my nose run that much. What was, behind my running nose, (which quite often ran more than I did) was what she was feeding me and my sisters along with her and my dad. It was the same stuff that she was raised on and that she fed her siblings when she cooked for them. It was a food that didn't use to be nearly as dangerous as it is now.

Now, this food is severely tainted, courtesy of Monsanto in the US, Syngenta in Europe and the rest of the world, And Bayer is now merged with Monsanto. What does a drug company want with a crop seed company? Do they want to make sure our food stays tainted? Fortunately yet, not all sources of our food supply are as tainted as those of grains, sugar, and potatoes. But usually, what you find that isn't tainted, isn't far from tainted food, unless you can find an organic dairy that feeds its cows uncontaminated grass or alfalfa. This is why I live mostly on what I can get from my local organic dairy where their cows are pasture fed with no antibiotics, ever used on them.

Since I've been following this pattern in my diet, I've not gotten ill yet. I haven't had any headaches, stomach aches, colds, flues, or any kind of discomfort. This, to me, is what your food is supposed to provide, a healthy body to fight off illnesses. I don't buy snacks as I don't hunger for them, Actually, I don't get that hungry due to my body being in ketosis all of the time. It's those nasty carbs that drive your hunger, forcing you into a cycle of dependence that doesn't let up until you give them up. I've learned that the longer I can go each day without food in my stomach, the more growth hormones I can manufacture to keep my body healthier and my brain sharper. This is the price I pay for my health. While you're buying your bread, pasta, pastries, donuts, and crackers, I'm keeping my stomach empty to build up growth hormones in my body. It's amazing how easy it is without the grains and sugar in my diet.

What price are you paying for your health? Do you ever get headaches? Ever, get stomach aches? Do your mosquito bites flare up from inflammation? I don't get mosquito bites. Since they're attracted to the glycolysis on your breath and I don't transform carbs in my body to fat, I eat the fat directly, I don't smell like glucose to the mosquitoes, so they leave me alone. This was a benefit I didn't expect but it sure is appreciated.

How much do you spend each month for aspirin, Advil, or Aleve to quell your pains? How much do you spend on anti-inflammatories? How much do you spend on antacids or stomach medicine like Pepto Bismol? How much do you spend every time you go to the doctor to get a prescription? Are you on Chemotherapy? How much does that cost? Do you take blood pressure medication? It's not hard to see how much the pharmaceutical industry is making off this ruse. How much of that is your money? A lot of it was mine. I had to pay it. The pain was just too much to live with. I just couldn't stand the misery I was in pain with, most of the time. They got plenty of my money. I remember how much I loved the corn chips, snack crackers, soda, and everything else that drives the pain. It's no wonder I had to pay so much for the drugs to buy my relief.

When you multiply this by the number of people in our nation and the world who've all fallen victim to this ruse, you can see why statistics of all major diseases are on the rise. Glyphosate spraying is also on the rise. Are you starting to see the correlation? There definitely is one.

Monsanto makes money from the sales of the Roundup that their contracted farmers have to spray. They're contracting as many as they can as I type this page. After they profit from the sales of their Roundup, they profit from the sale of the same chemicals to their sister industry the pharmaceutical industry. They use these same chemicals to isolate control of their other drugs to enable them to work in more specialized ways. They're usually used in heart medications and cancer medications, both conditions which are caused by ingestion of their food. Does this sound like something that should be legal? Unfortunately, it is, and Monsanto, now owned by Bayer, takes advantage it, substantially.

That should alarm you. Bayer a German-owned pharmaceutical company, now owns Monsanto, owner of 15 crop seed companies, all selling crop seed to farmers for food to feed you. "Control the food and you can control the people." That was according to Stalin. Your food, America, is now controlled by a German corporation, and if you feel comfortable with that, I'll come back in 5 years and ask again, if you're still alive.

This is the danger that's been imposed on our society, at the expense of corporate profit. Your lives will be endangered once Bayer has full control. But they can only control you if you remain victim into this ruse, so my advice to you is to avoid the pain, avoid the ruse, avoid the bread and sugars.

Unless you really like keeping profits high for the pharmaceutical corporations, the chemical corporations that supply the pharmaceutical companies, you probably feel like I do. It's time to end their influence in the health of America. So far, it's been disastrous. No regulation would have almost been better, but we get to live with what was given to us, whether it was in our best interest, or not, and in this case, it wasn't.

This ruse is an ultimate ploy to take your money, as much as possible, for the control of pain, for the treatment of cancer, heart disease, inflammation and a myriad of major diseases, all that have the power to kill. The problem is that they kill ever so slowly, it's painful and expensive, very expensive and that's why this ruse stays in place, taking your money. That makes, feeding your addiction your most expensive habit. As long as you continue to buy into this ruse, your expenses won't end, until you die. Then, your family might be on the hook for your death or life's expenses, which are going to be plenty if your health demands it. That conjures the question, how much did you spend to get your body in that condition that you needed all those medications? How much did you spend on all the bread products that you've eaten all your life? How much did you spend on beer and alcohol? Those are concentrated sugars. That's why it makes you so loopy.

However much you enjoyed spending, making yourself sick, you'll spend 4 times that amount, trying to keep yourself healthy, which you won't be able to do, if you're relying on drugs to treat your pain. If you want to play our medical industry's game of treatment, you're going to be stuck doing drugs for the rest of your life, which will ultimately be truncated by about 20-30 years. That's the nature of glycolysis and a carb diet that prompts that glycolysis that initiates the glycation that's at the root of all modern major disease.

THE CARBS YOU CRAVE FROM ALL YOUR THE GRAINS

ARE RESPONSIBLE FOR ALL OF YOUR ACHES AND PAINS,

IT'S SO UNFORTUNATE THAT OUR BREAD
IS WHAT'S MAKING MOST OF US PREMATURELY DEAD.
AND IT DOES COME FROM WHAT IT DOES TO YOUR HEAD
BY POLLUTING YOUR BLOOD WITH GLYCATION'S DREAD
TO FILL YOUR BODY WITH INFLAMMATION AND PAIN
RATHER THAN GIVING YOU NOURISHMENT
FROM GLYPHOSATED GRAIN
WHICH HINDERS BODY AND ALSO BRAIN
TO RESTORE YOUR HEALTH
AND GIVE YOU FOOD THAT BRINGS YOU WEALTH
AS FOR DIABETES, THERE IS A CURE
THANKS TO DR. DAVIS, THAT'S NOW SURE
THAT WHAT WE'VE BEEN EATING IS FAR FROM CLEAR
OF THE DANGERS OF DIABETES, OBESITY, AND CANCER
THE ONLY WAY OUT IS TO COMPLETELY ABSTAIN
FROM ANY KIND OF CONSUMPTION OF ANY KIND OF GRAIN
IT'S SAD, I KNOW, CAUSE I LOVE IT TOO
BUT I BROKE MY ADDICTION JUST LIKE YOU CAN TOO
KNOWING JUST WHAT THIS BREAD'S DONE TO ME
HAS OPENED MY EYES TO A NEW ETERNITY
MINE IS NOT FINITE LIKE THOSE STILL ON THE GRAINS
MINE IS NOW MY LIFE, THAT I LEAD WITHOUT PAINS
YOURS CAN BE THAT LIFE IF YOU WISH IT TO BE
TO LIVE YOUR LIFE WITHOUT PAIN LET YOURSELF BE
COMPLETELY FREE
IT IS YOUR CHOICE AS YOU WILL ULTIMATELY SEE
TO CONTINUE YOUR DIET OF GRAINS THAT WILL ULTIMATELY
COST YOU, MEDICALLY, FAR MORE MONETARILY
JUST TO STAY PAIN-FREE
WHICH WILL ULTIMATELY
TAKE YOUR LIFE PREMATURELY.
THIS DOESN'T HAVE TO BE AN ULTIMATUM,
YOU DON'T EVEN HAVE TO TAKE ME VERBATIM

JUST REMEMBER IT'S SOMETHING THAT'S SO VERY PLANE
IS COMPELLING YOU EAT ALL THOSE GRAINS
OF POLLUTION THAT RUNS IN THE BLOOD OF YOUR VEINS.
YOUR HUNGER CYCLE IS YOUR GAUGE OF THIS
THE MORE YOU HUNGER, THE MORE THAT'S AMISS
THE POLLUTION THAT YOU INSIST ON ADDING TO,
TO SATISFY YOUR BRAIN,
IT'S THIS SAME POLLUTION THAT CREATES ALL YOUR PAIN
IT'S ALSO THIS FOOD THAT YOU LOVE
THAT'S EATING UP YOUR BRAIN
BUT YOU'LL NEVER KNOW UNTIL YOU
GIVE IT UP THIS "GOOD FOOD" AND THROW IT DOWN THE DRAIN,
THEN, CAN YOU CHANGE YOUR ATTITUDE
TO A GOOD MOOD, BY EATING GOOD FOOD
THAT'S VOID OF THE CURSE OF THE DOUBLE FISTED PURSE.
I'LL BE THE FIRST TO ADMIT THAT IT ISN'T EASY
TO ABSTAIN FROM THIS GRAIN THAT'S MADE ME SO QUEASY
BUT AFTER I DID IT THE FREEDOM I FELT
WAS SO LIBERATING TO MY BRAIN
THAT MY MIND'S GOT NEW WEALTH
THE SECOND BEST THING IS THE IMPROVEMENT TO MY HEALTH
AS IT KEEPS ME FROM ENLARGING THE LOT BEHIND MY BELT
NOW, LIFE IS SO EASY FOR ME, ANSWERS COME SO LIBERALLY
THAT I'M CAUGHT WONDERING HOW I MANAGED BEFORE MY CHANGE
FOR EVERYTHING IT DID TO MY LIFE IT DID REARRANGE
NOW THAT MY THINKING IS CLEARER I'VE COME TO REALIZE
THAT MY FUTURE HAS CHANGED TO OPEN MY EYES
TO BRING ME THE GAIN I'VE LACKED ALL MY YEARS
TO SEE THE REAL BLAME FOR WHAT'S BROUGHT ALL MY TEARS
THAT AN INDUSTRY BUILT TO INCREASE OUR PAINS
HAS DEVELOPED IN THE WORLD OF THE GROWING OF GRAINS.

IX
Restaurant Ruse of the
Glucose Ruse Blues

Why it's such a hard addiction to break!

My father loved eating out. He and Mom enjoyed a different restaurant every day and I think that, ultimately may have been what was responsible for taking her. Had Dad known that, he would have done differently, I know. But he didn't know that institutional food suppliers don't supply ingredient lists for all of the foods they offer their clients, the restaurants, and stores in town.

I think this is what hurt Mom the most, because the first thing you get, often before you even get your menu, is your appetizer. This appetizer is supposed to heighten your appetite for when they take your order. It does that by making you hungrier. That's why your appetizer is always, either bread or bread coated, and this is your hidden indication of what you're there for, to feed your addiction.

Mom loved bread. He arm was magnetically attracted to those appetizers, every time they put them on the table. That appetizer was her immediate fix, for her addiction. Her addiction ultlmately killed her in the summer of 2016, one month after I published my first book, *It's Time to Curb Your Carbs to Save Your Life and Keep Your Dignity*. Yeah, I know that's a long title, but it was my first book and I just wanted to get it published, to give my mother a chance to read it, to hopefully save her from her third fight with breast cancer. This time, it metastasized in her bones. Breast cancer in the bones? How can that be? She was told, it was the same cancer that took her breasts, the two times she fought it before, but this time, it came back in her bones. I think it was the anger I expressed in my book that may have helped take my mother's life, forcing me to query my decision to share it with her. I can only imagine how she felt, reading it, experiencing my anger for her failure in controlling her addiction. That tells me, this addiction exists in the blood, as it's an addiction that affects the brain as well as the body.

The cancer is the exactly same, as it exists in the blood, no matter where it goes. That tells me it does exist everywhere, just like inflammation does, it has to be the inflammation that's causing the cancer. Control the inflammation, control the cancer. The nice thing about this, is that it controls the heart disease too. And dementia, of any source, gets controlled as well. How great is this? Three major diseases, down the tubes, just from a change in diet. No drugs necessary. WOW!

But, to get back to who supplies your meal, when you eat out. In our community, there are two suppliers that I knew of. When I was in that business, I was never offered an ingredient list for anything they offered for wholesale. That leaves a lingering question in my mind, how does anyone know what they're eating when they eat out?

The problem with this question is the answer, there's only one answer to this question, they don't. I found out the hard way the other day when I went with a friend to a restaurant and got some hidden grains in my food, in the dish I ordered. I thought I ordered nothing but protein, but hidden in some of that protein was a filler. That filler had to have been wheat. (The restaurant had run out of ground sausage and had to substitute a broken sausage patty, to put in my omelet.) The sausage patty needs something to keep the sausage together and that was the filler that got me. That was another lesson that I've had to learn the hard way, 'cause I don't like mosquito bites. As my friend said, "It had to be something of that nature". I don't know exactly what it was they snuck in there. I just know that I don't get mosquito bites unless there's glucose in my system. I got a mosquito bite after coming home from going out to eat the other day with my friend. If I got bit, something put that glucose in my system without me knowing it. I never eat anything that has any carbohydrate in it knowingly, so it must have been snuck into my food at the restaurant.

That is a good reason as any, to only eat in at home, where you know what you're eating because you prepared it and you read the ingredients on the package or you cleaned the produce or meat yourself. You don't have those luxuries when you eat out. You're relying on the source where that restaurant gets their food from, that what they're feeding you is 100% safe to eat.

The biggest problem with this gets into the food the restaurant loves to feed you first, as soon as you walk in the door. That's bread because bread makes you hungry. All bread they serve gets desiccated two weeks, before harvest, to guarantee the inclusion of glyphosate in your diet. Every restaurant knows that bread makes you hungrier. So does my dad, yet he continued playing their game, not knowing what the underlying damage that hunger cycle was doing to him, my mom and our family. Unfortunately, It took my mother a year last summer while she was fighting cancer for the third time. All because she couldn't give up her love of bread.

Couple that with the fact the 95% of all resaurant fare is industrially grown, which happens to be the most heavily glyphosated crops, so they can be purchased cheaply. This lowers the bottom line for the restaurant. but It shortens your infection time, in doing so.Fast food restaurants are the worst perpetrators of this part of the restaurant ruse of the Glucose Ruse Blues.

Does that mean that bread creates cancer? Yeah. it does. Doesn't that mean that you shouldn't eat bread? Yeah, it does. Unless you can give up your love of bread, your fate will be the same or close to it. I'm sorry, but it's written in the law of digestion and there's nothing you can do about it, except to give up your love of bread.

The reason the bread is so bad is because of the glycation it creates, plus the fact that Monsanto has ramped up the glycation by desiccating (spraying glyphosate *Roundup* weed killer on the entire crop two weeks before it's harvested), virtually guaranteeing that it ends up in your diet so it can inflict all the harm that the poison can inflict (and it inflicts plenty).

Grains are desiccated 2 weeks before harvest, to quickly ripen the plant for a higher yield. Ground crops get desiccated 3 days before harvest, to kill the ground weeds, for easier harvest. Do you think that might guarantee, it gets into your food? (Keep in mind, glyphosate goes to the root and foliage.)

Since the three enzymes that it inhibits the most, are tyrosine, tryptophan, and phenylalanine, all enzymes that influence fear, digestion, hunger, and sleep, and the fact that all grains get desiccated, it would seem to me that to stay away from any grain food is the only guaranteed way to stay away from disease, discomfort and extreme pain (the kind of pain that killed my mother).

GLYPHOSATE'S PAINS DRIVEN BY FAST FOOD'S CHAINS

Most industrial food grown in America is used for Restaurants including fast food chains, like McDonalds and Burger King. They both grow all their food industrially, which mean rampant use of glyphosate to make it cheap food. The cheapness wears off after you ingest it, when it makes you sick from the excess glyphosate.

Case in point, look at President Trump who admittedly buys a lot of his groceries at McDonalds. Look at his fear levels. They're off the charts.

How many people, these days, buy their groceries through the drive-thru window? How much glyphosate are they consuming on a daily basis? What influence does that have on our society and its fear levels? Can you see the correlation?

This fast food glyphosate ruse is the worst part of the restaurant ruse of the glucose ruse blues, and is quite possibly the most successful ruse this industry has going, challenging only the breakfast cereal ruse, which includes, the pastry ruse. How many people go out to eat? How many of those people ask for an ingredient list for the dishes they're served? How many of them know exactly what they're putting in their bodies? How many people know of the glyphosate, they eat with every donut or roll they take a bite of? Have you asked Dunkin Donuts how much they know about glyphosate? The kind that goes into every donut in the flour and sugar that they're made from?

I submit that none of them know. I submit that few of them even care. The last thing on their minds is the quality of the food they're about to ingest, they're concerned mostly about how it tastes, and how it's prepared. It's assumed that's it's safe to eat because it's coming from a restaurant. They have to serve safe food, don't they? Nobody wants food poisoning from a restaurant, so that's watched for religiously, but even the regulators are letting some food slip by, due to their ignorance of the truth. We realized that in the last chapter.

Much of this ignorance is due to the fact, the corporation controlling the lion's portion of your food supply, also controls the regulatory agency, that's supposed to be monitoring this industry, virtually guaranteeing that you will be poisoned if you eat their food. The biggest problem with this is, you will never know you're being poisoned until it's too late to do anything about it except to fight the pain that your disease will bring and this is exactly where this industry wants you.

They want you in pain, ready to buy their newest pain killing NSAIDs or opioids. I know. I've been there. I've been there many times over the last 30 years and I do not wish to visit there ever again and this is why; NSAIDs create liver and kidney cancer. It's in the nature of the way the body filters the chemicals to clean them out of the body. They have a tendency to put undue strain on these organs, that wouldn't be necessary if they were never needed in the first place.

That brings us to the primary question; if the pain never existed in the first place, would you need the pain-killing drugs? That brings us to the second question; how do you avoid creating the pain? And that brings us to the key answer, don't eat that which creates the pain, the glucose in all carbs. That brings us to a very simple solution, don't eat grains of any sort. Don't eat cereal grains or legume grains, they're all poisoned.

I think Mom always wanted to be a good mom more than anything in the world and that's probably why she was such a good cook and baker. She assumed that all good moms had to be good cooks and bakers, as that's what she was taught in her childhood. Because her father died when she was 8, her mother had to find a man to take care of them in 1939, the end of the depression, when a woman had to rely on men for their economic survival and well-being. I believe that she thought the better cook and baker she was, the better mom she was. I also think that it was from recommendations from our government on how to be a good parent, that drove her behavior.

I'm thankful that Dad wanted to be the father that was taken away from him when he was an infant by what was Child Protective Services at that time in 1932 when my dad turned 1 year old. He was taken away from his father when his mother abandoned him while still an infant. Since his father couldn't take care of him while working or looking for work, the state took my father and his siblings and put all 4 of them in foster homes. This was when my father was separated from the rest of his family, as he was born in a different county than they were. This is also what allowed my mother to meet my father.

Mom wanted to be the best wife and mother she could be, I think because her mother worked most of the time. I can't remember a time when Grandma wasn't working. Grandpa, on the other hand, stayed around the farm and ran his country Watkins store. But, what I want to point out is that my mother fed me what she was fed herself, by her mother, who was, in turn, feeding her what she grew up on, the food my great-grandmother cooked and baked.

This is why my grandmother died of Alzheimer's disease and why my mother died of cancer. I don't remember Grandpa, without diabetes. He was the first to die. I've lost the only grandfather, I remember, past 3 years old, and 2 uncles, both of which died of heart disease. This is why my aunt has had bouts with breast cancer. This is why my sister is diabetic and my father pre-diabetic and takes medicine that's altering his hormones to not function properly. (Medicines have a tendency to do that.)

This is what ultimately leads only to more and more medications and ultimately sucks you into a cycle of dependence that's no different than that of another addiction that starts this whole cycle. That is the addiction of the Glucose Ruse.

There is no way to way to get away from it as we're all born into it. It's what all of our mothers' fed us while we were fetuses. This simple practice makes this addiction completely involuntary, which means that it's been inflicted upon us, without our knowledge or consent. When one thinks about the ramifications of this, it's astounding. It means that all the disease this diet creates has been involuntarily imposed upon us, due to our addictions and admiration for its lures. That is what I call a celebration of addiction. 98% of us are guilty of it. I don't know of anyone who hasn't had birthday cake.

By realizing this, it's easier to get an idea of just how much this permeates our society and worse yet, commerce. It's the commerce side of it that drives all disease and disorder, as well as all terrorism as it's the hunger cycle created by the addiction to sugar that's at the base of all fear and subsequent, terrorism. The disease, disorder, and terrorism would still exist without the prevalence of sugar that exists today, but it wouldn't exist to the extent that it exists now.

That's due to the rampant glyphosation all grains go through now, increasing everyone's fear levels. Due to the desiccation and liberal use of this enzyme inhibiting pesticide, our society has displayed a massive amount of reaction to the glyphosation in the increases of in cancer, heart disease, dementia, phobias, and even autism. Every one of these disorders has increased right alongside the use of glyphosate. Unfortunately though, due to the regulatory agency being controlled by this same industry, they chose to remain completely ignorant of this revelation (even though it's over 30 years old).

It just wouldn't have been profitable to heed this message. What was learned, was that this could be used to profit off of this addiction, and profit they did. All at the cost of the consumer's health. The consumer in this context includes all of those who need to buy groceries. This brings another unwanted addiction to those who choose to participate in this ruse. It leads directly to a never-ending cycle of drug use, just to end the pain. That makes this industry completely responsible for your pain, discomfort, and death due to their imposition of this addiction on all who buy into it.

If you're looking for the real reason the opioid epidemic exists? You don't need to look any further. This is your reason. End this cycle, you can end that cycle and all other addictive ones with it. They're all based in this cycle of hunger, fear, anger and pain. (They just seem to go together.)

Yet, this industry controls the agency that is supposed to regulate it. And regulation it needs, as the basis for this industry is chemical in nature and it has engineered its influence to spread their poison as wide as possible. This is how it gets into your food if you eat at a restaurant or buy your groceries at a grocery store. This is how they force you into a cycle of dependence on one of their other industries, the pharmaceutical industry. I know. I was there. Just 7 years ago.

That's when I gave them all up and I never felt better since. Initially, my weight came off, and that set up my body and mind so I could do away with my pain, without drugs. The lack of grains in my diet has done wonders of reducing the chronic levels of my pain to less than half of what they were before, but I still have to deal with break-thru pain, which this deals with very well. Of everything I tried over 20 years of fighting chronic pain, this works better than anything I've tried, except for acupuncture. And often, that was iffy, depending on the protocol used.

The choice I made, you can make too, to eliminate your pains. It's completely up to you, you can quit the bread and break your addiction, or you can continue to get sick. Don't look to the health industry or the medical industry to eliminate your pain. It's in their best interest to add to it, to insure their own bottom line. Why would they want to help you, at their expense? That's why this whole industry would rather, this information doesn't get out.

This is how these industries operate to expand their influence and power. It's all done at your expense. If you don't feel like a sap right now, you should because you are one, if you take part in it. They would rather keep it quiet to keep the secret to themselves. This is how they take your money. It's how they used to take mine until I got smart and quit eating, their invitation to my blues. Fortunately, you have that same choice, to continue eating their ruse or wizen up and stop the pain.

IT'S IN THIS RESTAURANT RUSE

THAT YOU PAY MOST OF YOUR DUES

DUE TO YOUR IGNORANCE THEY USE

TO BRING YOU MOST OF WHAT YOU'LL RUE

TO CREATE YOUR BLUES

X

THE POWER OF FASTING
THE OLDEST SUREST PATH TO HEALTH

Don't Be The Patsy by Buying into their Ruse
Learn the Power of Fasting to Quickly End Your Blues

For as far back as 500BC, physicians have used fasting as a means to find the way back to health by a simple and inexpensive manner in which one could actually heal themselves from virtually any of the modern diseases that have plagued man since the dawn of civilization. For me, it's easy to see the correlation of the emergence of modern diseases with the gradual increase of consumption of einkorn wheat, the precursor to our modern strains of wheat.

From Emmer, (one of the first domesticated strains) to Durum Semolina, which is little higher in gluten, yet, it's still considered a weak wheat, (the wheat doesn't rise as well as it holds the dough together to hold the pasta shape) to Winter Red, Spelt, and other bread wheat or common wheat that are higher in gluten, have been used for bread for thousands of years because they rise better. All wheat has an extreme tendency to create glycation more so today than it ever did in the past, due to genetic modifying for extreme glyphosation. Today's forms of highly modified wheat act nothing like the strains from thousands of years ago as today's *highly domesticated strains of wheat cannot survive in the wild.* That's according to Wikipedia and that's due to their inability to disperse their seeds, insuring, they can make their grain, more glycative than it has ever been throughout our history as a species. This is your first clue as to why fasting works.

Monsanto has made certain of that through their genetic modifying to create ender seeds that won't pollinate so a farmer has no seed for next year's crop forcing them to buy GMO seed from Monsanto. (GMO by itself is not dangerous. It's what the modifying allows the farmer to do that makes it dangerous and that's to spray it with Roundup. Their seed is genetically modified to handle applications of the glyphosate herbicide.) This is the wheat that Monsanto is forcing their farmers to grow for your cereal, bread, and snacks. The same exists in the cornfields as well, contaminating every corn chip that you eat. (When was the last time you ate Mexican food?)

And we haven't talked about soy yet. You can't find hardly any processed food that doesn't have soy in it. We're talking about wheat right now which was originally cultivated in the Fertile Crescent starting, 9,000 years ago, probably by the Natufians. around, approximately the same time that modern disease started showing up in the bones of the remains of the people. This is a clear indication of the glycation that wheat was responsible for even then, even as slow as the einkorn wheat is to digest (which slows the progression of glycation). The glycation existed then as it does now, only it took it much longer to manifest. Today, it manifests itself immediately (as soon as it touches your tongue) and this is due to the fast dissolving gluten flour that's used for bread and pastries as well as pasta and cereal.

Remember the 5,000 year old iceman, from chapter 4 and his signs of atherosclerosis and arthritis? Remember what they found in his stomach? This is your indication that it glycated then. It just glycates more now as the grain has changed immensely in the last 7,000 years. As this food increased in prevalence in our diet, the rates of disease increased, as it's these grains that have always generated disease. They generate it so slowly that it's never noticed until it's too late or you stop eating it. This points to the value of fasting and why fasting is so important to the health of anyone on this type of carbohydrate diet.

This is why fasting has always cured disease. 98% of all disease is a direct result of our diet. With that being said, it's easy to see why removing everything damaging from our diet is going to heal the damage caused by keeping those foods in the diet. Fasting produces such good results it's been the subject of over 20,000 studies on PMC in the NLM at the NIH. (PMC has reports from across the world. Pubmed has 590 reports from studies done in the US alone.) It's that important, yet what has your doctor shared with you about this life-saving course of intervention?

Your doctor comes into your appointed meeting with his/her prescription tablet in hand ready to prescribe pharmaceuticals. (Now. if your insurance is like mine and linked to my healthcare - where they digitally prescribe my medications - it's a laptop that affords them more latitude in their diagnosis. I sometimes see a primary care physician who still carries a prescription pad with him everywhere he goes, but then, he has drug reps going in and out of his office all the time, so to speak.) Their whole intent is to prescribe drugs for your ailments, which are more than likely caused by the ingestion of grain foods. Prescribing drugs is the way they're trained to treat patients, not with recommendations of diet. (Monsanto wouldn't allow that to take place as they have far more control over your life than what you could ever believe.)

That's exactly why fasting is so healthy. It removes the worst of the toxins in our bodies that are built up from the diets of bread, wheat, and grain-based products, and doesn't put more toxins back in with the prescribed drugs. Those grain products also happen to be the most addictive, which is what makes them the hardest to give up. The addictive nature of sugar, at its worst, is displayed in this manner (when it drives pharmaceuticals). When one fasts, they give up the sugars that are doing all the glycating and it's this glycation that is at the root of all disease and this is why going without this food is so healthy.

It also sets your body up for future health by resetting the hormonal structure in your body. This is mostly the result of your hormones transitioning to a starvation mode of survival, where the Ghrelin your stomach releases, sends this growth hormone throughout your body allowing it to do its magic in repairing damage and extending cell life where cell death took place before. (This is directly due to the carbohydrate influence in the diet, creating glycation.)

It's the elimination of glycation that initially brings back a resemblance of health but that's not what brings future health. It's the breaking of an addiction. This addiction is built into our society so much, It starts in our prenatal body and continues through the first year of life and then on. (This is due to the prevalence of sugar and high fructose corn syrup in baby foods, formula, and infant medicines.) The prenatal starts with mama's diet before you're born, if your mother ate carbs, you got them before you were born.

But that only explains why you're dependent. It doesn't explain how to break the dependence. That's with fasting and the keto diet, the diet our ancestors were on throughout our evolution. The keto diet involves fasting as part of the diet, making it much easier to maintain. (There's no hunger, once you break the addiction.) Fasting does that by sending your body into ketosis.

According to Wikipedia; "in the early 20th century around 1911; Bernarr Macfadden, an American exponent of physical culture, popularized the use of fasting to restore health. His disciple, the osteopathic physician Hugh Conklin, of Battle Creek, Michigan, began to treat his epilepsy patients by recommending fasting. Conklin conjectured that epileptic seizures were caused when a toxin, secreted from the Peyer's patches in the intestines, was discharged into the bloodstream. Conklin's fasting therapy was adopted by neurologists in mainstream practice. In 1916, a Dr. McMurray wrote to the New York medical journal claiming to have successfully treated epilepsy patients with a fast, followed by a starch-free and sugar-free diet, since 1912. In 1921, prominent endocrinologist. Rawle Geyelin reported his experiences to the American medical association convention. He had seen Conklin's success first-hand and had attempted to reproduce the results in 36 of his own patients. He achieved similar results despite only having studied the patients for a short time. He reported that three water-soluble compounds, β-hydroxybutyrate, acetoacetate and acetone (known collectively as ketone bodies), were produced by the liver in otherwise healthy people when they were starved or if they consumed a very low-carbohydrate, high-fat diet." The excess ketone bodies in the blood prompted this diet to be labeled a ketogenic diet.

According to PMC's report on Calorie Restriction (CR) or fasting, submitted; July 2010;

"Nevertheless, ongoing research continues to draw a more complete picture of CR at the molecular level, which may ultimately allow for the development of therapeutics that might be able to confer at least some of the health benefits of this dietary regimen."

With fasting being able to eliminate so many disorders, a path was sought to bring this form of healing to the mainstream by creating a diet to encourage fasting. Thus the ketogenic diet was born in 1921 through the efforts of Russel Wilder. According to Wikipedia;

"Russel Wilder, at the Mayo Clinic, built on this research and coined the term ketogenic diet to describe a diet that produced a high level of ketone bodies in the blood (ketonemia) through more emphasis on fat and a lack of almost all carbohydrates."

Fasting is the quickest manner in which to allow your body to go into ketosis, yet it may not be the easiest. Although on second thought, being the quickest way may make it the easiest. I went through two to three weeks of withdrawal because I couldn't give up all foods I loved to eat, all at once, to allow my body to go into ketosis in a few days.

I could have avoided 10 days of hunger and want, by fasting and only hunger, for something to eat, for a few days as that's what happens when you fast for a minimum of 3 days. A longer fast is more beneficial but the three days allows your body to respond by going into ketosis which is a fat burning mode.

It's this fat burning mode that encourages your body to make its own glucose, which is a much cleaner glucose than you get from the sugar you eat. It's a clean glucose made from your own glycogen or fat storage. Getting into ketosis quicker could allow you to convert your hormones quicker by starting your fat burning glucagon quicker, but continuing some carbs will only make the withdrawal more difficult as it will drop your body back out of ketosis. This was my problem and why my transition took so long. (Thankfully, they'll be no next time.)

Ketosis refers to acids in the body that are derived and used while in a state of low glucose in the blood. Because my body has been in a state of ketosis for the last 4 years, I feel qualified to speak about this lifestyle. I call it a lifestyle because it really is.

A carboholic's day is organized around meals. Not so, with someone in ketosis. It's a lifestyle completely different from the lifestyle of a carboholic. Carboholics require food every other hour or so, it's the law of glucose consumption, appetite follows glucose levels in the blood. It's that simple, blood sugar levels rise and satiety sets in, releasing hormones controlling feel-good emotions influencing behavior, sometimes unrecognizable behavior. But, that usually happens when the blood sugars fall again after a couple hours, releasing hormones of hunger, need and want. These hormones are completely different than the satiety hormones and have muchly different effects on the body, mostly influencing emotions like fear.

This is where carboholics do not have the advantage that ketonemiacs have. Ketonemiacs (those who have allowed their bodies to go into a state of ketosis) aren't controlled by their hormones, so they don't have to follow any hunger cycle. They're in full control of their hormones. This also means that they're in more control of their emotions because of that. I know that it doesn't sound like it's that big of a deal, but it's more important than you ever could imagine.

Remaining in a state of ketosis has allowed my body to regain that which was lost 31 years ago in a car accident that left me severely disabled because of a severe closed head injury, (It was the two strokes that were the most devastating.) It's become evident to me since I've been carb free and in a state of ketonemia or ketosis, how much our society is addicted to this drug (sugar/glucose/fructose) that does little more than to lead those who eat it to further drug use. Our food industrial complex sees to that by their advertising. I'm convinced it's because they're associated with the pharmaceutical industry. They used to be merged into one corporation that controlled the seed supply for the farmers as well as the pharmaceuticals that treated the pain and discomfort brought on by the products grown by the crop seed sold to the farmer to supply the grains for the snack foods everyone everywhere loves to eat. Now that Bayer purchased Monsanto, They clearly do. How trusting are you? Does this ruse sound like something you'd like to cruise, or would you rather lose it?

The unfortunate result of this love affair with those snack and comfort foods is what this diet brings, as its cost of this pleasure cruise. The price to be paid is in the discomfort that this food brings to all those who eat it, regardless of how much they eat. The food industry (Monsanto in particular) has a fortune invested in keeping you eating this deadly food. They've built an industry just to treat diabetes, with all the glucose meters and pumps out there, just so addicts can get their next fix. This is part of the trouble this industry goes to just to keep their addicts happy. I know now. I didn't 5 years ago when I was an addict.

The amount an addict consumes at each sitting, dictates how much damage it's going to do, but it's going to do damage. There is no way to avoid it. That's the way our digestion and metabolism works. That's why this addiction is by far, the worst addiction our society has to deal with. This addiction leads to every other addiction that we're actively fighting, including alcoholism, heroin and tobacco and even gambling. Yes, even gambling, as gambling is driven by the hunger cycle which is one of the biggest underlying influences of a carbohydrate diet. Hunger in this diet drives absolutely everything, even breathing, and because of that, eventually drugs. And yes, that does mean that the opioid epidemic is caused by a diet high in carbohydrates.

This is a cycle that I don't need. As a matter of fact, it's the last thing I need. The biggest reason I refuse to take any of these drugs anymore is due to the fact, all of them carry side effects, some major, some minor. Whether the side effects are major or minor, I don't want to experience any of them, anymore. I've had my fill of side effects, especially the ones that make my health worse, which is where most of these side effects should be classified. After living for twenty years needing to take massive amounts of opioids for my chronic severe pain, diuretics for my high blood pressure, antidepressants for the pain, and living with the side effects of not only the opioids, but every other drug they had me on, all twelve of them, I got fed up with it. I wasn't going to take it anymore as I just couldn't afford it. And I was only up to twelve medications. I have a friend who's on this diet, who's lowered his needs to thirteen daily medications from twenty-three. How many meds do you take every day? How many would you like to do without, if your health would allow? This is where fasting needs to replace doping. A change in diet will go much further than any drug and the cure lasts longer than any treatment.

I live by the theory that if the meds aren't needed in the first place, my health is going to be that much better. That is why I removed everything from my diet that I could, that is responsible for these horrendous diseases, requiring the need for these medications. By fasting, one can reach this healing state much quicker than I did, just by cutting my bread. Where it took me two weeks to get into full ketosis, by fasting I could have jump-started the state by starving my body, and then, gone on from there with my ketogenic diet to keep my body in this healing state. This is the advantage of fasting, it not only starts the healing from the beginning by putting your body in a starvation mode, it allows you to stay in that mode for the rest of your life. That one little option in itself is what's going to extend your life beyond 100 years. I can see where ultimately man will be able to extend its lifespan to over 150 years old. 100 years from now, when all mankind is on a ketogenic or paleo diet again, I can see the oldest people in the world living into their 180's, doubling today's average lifespan.

This can be easily obtained simply by allowing our bodies to heal themselves and not keep depending on drugs for the perception of healing, which ultimately brings nothing but more drug use, which ultimately is what ruins the liver and kidneys leading to all the cancers and disorders of the hepatic and renal systems. It's this drug dependence that driven by another dependence that we've all been born into. I hope that you're beginning to see how our drug addictions are driven by one thread that drives all modern diseases along with it. That one thread is what ties 100% of all cancers, 98% of all heart diseases, and 99.9 % of all dementia, all arthritis, all headaches and almost all stomachaches together. It's one substance that can be removed from the diet without any severe side effects. I shouldn't need to tell you what that substance is by now. You eat it every day. You live with the effects of addiction. Pain always comes with addiction. (That's what makes breaking the addiction so rewarding, limiting the pain cycle. Oh, what sweet bliss!)

The idea then is to limit to minuscule amounts, the foods that make up these addictive substances. You should know by now what these foods are, you eat them every morning, either in your coffee as creamer, in the toast you have, or the cereal you consume. You have it every lunch with your sandwich or burrito and with every dinner with your pasta and bread-rolls.

In a practice that disappeared toward the last half, of the last century, several families that would just put a plate of bread on the table every evening. This is the display of addiction, a full out need to satisfy the taste buds by dumping more and more sugar in the body, usually in the form of starchy carbs. I've also noticed that in those houses that served bread, there was always beer cans in the garbage indicating another addiction. If you remove this one addiction from our society, you remove all addictions, as this addiction to sugar and carbs is the foundation of all other addictions as they are all based on a hunger cycle which is the result of an addiction to sugar. Since the greed of hunger is at the base of all evil, wouldn't that put hunger at the root of all evil with it? That is where your danger lies, due to your carboholic addiction.

It's a little easier to see the connection, now, between terrorism and the fear that's created by your hunger cycle complicated with the massive amounts of glyphosate added to intentionally make you more afraid. What are you afraid of? Cancer? Heart disease? Alzheimer's in a relative? You know. they make medicine, for all of that, don't you?

I hope that you can see now, that it's this addiction to sugar and carbs that is driving the pharmaceutical industry, and that both industries are driven by the same people who have a major influence in the offices of the agencies that are supposed to regulate this industry, the FDA, and the USDA. With that kind of influence, there's only one way to fight it and that's to not buy into it. To not buy into it does require a diet of grain abstinence, though. That requires breaking the addiction and moving to, as ketogenic of a diet, as possible. The easiest manner to do this is to do a strict three day, water only, fast. The longer you can do it the better, but it must be at least 3 days with absolutely no food. **It's recommended to fast 1 day for every pound in weight, you want to lose, as fasting will allow you to lose a pound a day, to reach our optimum weight. The record is 60 lbs in 58 days.** (This man was extremely obese, over 350 lbs. That's why it's important to check with your doctor first, if you're on medications.)

All of the consumption of the grain industry's products is what's driving the pharmaceutical industry today, tomorrow, next year, and for the next 500 and beyond. If we don't put an end to this now, our society is doomed to suffer the consequences of a carbohydrate addiction that no one is responsible for. The greed of the grain industry combined with the ambition of the pharmaceutical industry has made us all carboholic slaves to the desires of these industries. It's these industries that are rewarding the most, from this arrangement. For me, it's scary, how much power we've given these industries, simply because we listen to their advertising. We've also let them take over the regulating agency that's supposed to control this industry. Because our health depends on it, we can't allow Monsanto to dictate how they are going to poison our food, so they can bolster the profits of the pharmaceutical industry.

Not knowing what you put in your body can cost you your life. It is costing you your life if you eat carbs. Those who listen to the advertising and are influenced by it, fall prey to that influence and become their slaves for life or until they quit consuming the grains. There's very little difference between carbolism and alcoholism, except that it's pretty much forced upon us, in our baby food. Mamas, feed your babies your own milk if you want them to be healthy.

I know what you're thinking right now, what are all the foods involved in this addiction? The list is enormous and that's why this is such a dangerous addiction. This industry has virtually forced us to celebrate this addiction. It involves every one of our holidays, with the holiday season being the worst. Every celebration involves some form of sugar. From the Sugar Bowl to the Tostido's Fiesta Bowl, our celebration is never-ending. Just after the "holiday season" comes Valentine's Day barely a month later. Then, comes Easter and spring break. Are you beginning to understand why this addiction is our worst? With all the celebrating we need, to keep this addiction, how do you change tradition without changing the world? The quickest way that I know is to organize an international health weekend, for 3 days, where everyone goes keto to heal their diseases and give their bodies a chance to go into ketosis, the ever healing state of metabolism.

The nicest advantage of this diet is the amount of control it gives you over your own emotions. You may think that you control your emotions right now, but I can tell you with full confidence, if you're on a carb diet, you have little control over your emotions. They're controlled by, more than anything, what you eat because what you eat controls your hunger cycle and it's your hunger cycle that drives every other cycle your body goes through. Since your hunger cycle is controlled by your hormones (mostly leptin and ghrelin), it's these hormones that are controlling your emotions. You know this every time you crave that bagel or biscotti. Once you bite into it, your saliva starts digesting that instantly gratifying food to give you that *mmmgood* feeling, that instantly hits your brain, even before you can swallow it. This is your first sign of addiction and dependence that only gives you the perception that you have control of your own emotions. It's this cycle that's in control of your emotions. As much as you try to control them, too often they have a tendency to slip out of your control and back into theirs.

Anyone who can't control their emotions entirely by themselves is a slave to their own hormones. This makes every carboholic a slave to their emotions and therefore a slave to these industries. This displays the dependence of the hunger cycle and the carb diet that drives that hunger cycle. You may not classify these as emotions, but I submit that they actually are. Satiety is defined as the state of being satisfied. If that is not an emotion, as it expresses feelings of calmness and security, I don't know what is. Hunger, on the other hand, is defined as a strong desire. Is not that an emotion? These emotions are controlled by both leptin and ghrelin, which ultimately are controlled by the grain industry, more than anything else. This is the ruse I refuse to take part in. I can't afford this trap anymore. The only way out for our society, is to break the hold of this industry, to let them know that we're not going to stand for this kind of abuse. To go ketogenic in your diet is the best way you can get yourself to everlasting health.

With emotions being controlled by our hormonal balance like this, it's easy to see how carbs could influence that balance. For this to not have an effect on our behavior is beyond comprehension. When you combine the drive of an addiction (which is what we're talking about) with the advertisements promoting that addiction, how can it not have an effect on our health and ultimately our society? That is why I make the statement that this cycle has to change. If it doesn't cease, our health as a society will never get better. There's never been a better time for a cure, and that cure is a ketogenic diet, not only for each and everybody to be as healthy as possible, but also to regain the health of our society, as a whole. Can you imagine a world where everyone not only controls their own emotions but they're in control of their emotions? (That includes reactions.)

Let's go back to addiction, though, for you may still not consider this an addiction. I understand few caught in an addiction can recognize that addiction when they're feeding it because the addiction has ways of hiding itself. You can ask anyone who has to have at least one beer a day. They're not addicted to their beer, as far as they're concerned, yet they have to have it. And often they don't even drink more than just one. But they still have to have that one. That is what makes it an addiction. The body can and does live much better without beer, so it's not a substance the body requires to survive. Yet the beer drinker needs that daily beer to satisfy their addiction. To go without, many times causes more problems because of the work your hormones are doing on your emotions and worse yet your actions by controlling how receptors work in your brain. That makes it a natural thing that you need to do, and not an addiction, to appease that desire to drink the beer. This can also create physical distress, if the need isn't met. This is how addiction works and it happens to carboholics too. I know I am a carboholic. The desire for sweets is still with me. It's a last refuge of my addiction. It's something that I get to fight for the rest of my life.

The fact of the matter is, if you were fed baby food, you've been fed carbs, on the premise that this food is healthy to eat. Actually, you've been sold that this is the only healthy food to eat. Fault has been found in every other type of nutrition except grains, until recent history. For more than 60 years, we've been told to eat grains. Thirty years ago, they said whole grains are healthy. They still say "whole grains are healthy", yet according to all the studies I've seen out of the hundreds I've looked at, nothing about this food is safe to ingest, leaving me to wonder why do they still recommend it. Remember the whole Einkorn grain that Ogli ate, 5000 years ago? Remember what they found in his arteries? When I look at who controls the FDA, the USDA and what interest they have in their industrial farming, it becomes pretty clear whose influence this is, controlling what we eat. This simple little act of feeding your baby formula laced with sugars to get them to eat it has addicted them and you to a lifetime of dependence. It addicted me. Even though I broke the addiction, I'm still affected by what control it did have over me. That's exactly why I'm pleading with you, don't let it control you. I can virtually guarantee that you won't like the end results. Whether they come late or soon, they always come.

When I think about this, my first response is to get angry, for I never asked for this nor could I ever wish for it, or wish it upon anyone else. Yet, there is an industry that is committed to not only continuing this pattern, their goal is to increase its scope. You can see this in all the advertising. This is your grain industry pushing this celebration of this addiction and you're buying into it every time you feed your carb diet, by buying all your snacks, pasta, cereal, soft drinks, and beer, just for starters. I'd go on with the rest but space limits that list in this book. You can find it in both my first and second books, *It's Time for a Cure* and *Time for the Ultimate Cure.*

Your best guide is to use the glycemic index as your guide for what foods that are safe to eat or not. It's the general consensus that you should keep your foods lower than 50 on the glycemic index. My contention is to keep carbs out of your diet completely and let your body make its own glucose. The reason you want to keep your blood glucose low is to avoid the hunger cycle. The hunger cycle is emotionally the worst manifestation of a carb diet. As it controls your emotions, it controls your actions and reactions. This is an undeniable truth. You know it as well as I do. You feel it every time you taste that divine taste when you bite into it, mmm how good it is.

This is where you need to ask yourself, what is it you crave most? If what you crave has any carbohydrate in it, then that's your first indication that you're addicted. What kind of carb you crave, quite often tells how bad your addiction is. One wouldn't think that a hamburger could be a sign of addiction, but actually when you think about the taste you crave, it's a combination of everything including the bun, which happens to be the addictive ingredient in the hamburger. Everything else in the hamburger is healthy. It's just the gluten in the bun that's so addictive. I wouldn't doubt that they use extra high gluten bread dough for the buns used for these sandwiches, as it's more addictive, due to the high gluten content. I know they use high gluten bread dough for making pizza dough because it needs to rise, and the more the gluten the better it rises. That makes it taste better, but it also makes it more addictive. That's why when you're at one of these restaurants, most everyone there is overweight. They're there because they crave that high gluten bread dough. You get it in both pizzas and fast food hamburgers. This is how they make you repeat customers. It's the high gluten bread flour that's the most addictive, due to it having the most glyphosate in it.

If you think my assessment is wrong, just try eating your favorite hamburger between to slices of lettuce. The taste is completely different. Most fast food restaurants offer low carb sandwiches but few order them. The only ones that I know of who order them are those who suffer from celiac disease. I believe that all of us suffer somewhat from celiac disease. I think that there are only a very few that can get through life without showing or suffering the effects of a carb diet....especially an excessive carb diet as is the case with most people worldwide today. The reason you crave the taste of the hamburger is because of the high gluten bread dough the buns are made from because it's that bun that raises your blood glucose as soon as it hits your tongue. Therein lies the addictive nature of glucose, the constant tug on your hunger cycle. It's caused by the foods you eat if you're on a carb diet. When you stop to think about it, you know it, as well as I. You just need to do something about it, as I did, six years ago, and then again four years ago when I went complete keto. It took me three years to go completely keto. You can do it in one month if you've got the guts to do a three day fast. I didn't and I may have suffered because of it. I guess I was still persuaded to eat the carbs even after I gave up the bread. If I had to do it over again, I'd fast, to go keto. The adjustment is a lot quicker. The adjustment is equivalent to breaking the addiction. What do you think they're advertising when they show you those commercials for pizza and their soft drinks, fruit drinks, cereals, bread, pasta, pastries, candy, etc, etc? They're selling you that mmm feeling of dependence and addiction. It's that feeling you get as soon as your favorite food hits your tongue and makes you go "oh, I needed that". That's the same feeling a junkie feels when he gets his latest fix.

They're using your emotions to control your behavior. That's because they can. They already control your hormones and it's your hormones that control your emotions. Is it any wonder that so many are addicted? Our food industry has done their absolute best to sell you their goods, and that means playing to your emotions in order to sell you that great taste that's going to bring you oh so much discomfort, pain, and disease. If you had known that this would happen to any one of your kids, you'd do everything in your power to change it. You do have the power to change it, every time you go to the store. Read the label of everything you buy. If it contains sugar, wheat, corn, soy or grains at all, don't buy it. If you do, you'll be buying a lifetime of pain and discomfort for your family. The problem here is that there is so much of it that's hidden, in almost all of our processed food that it's hard to tell exactly where it's at. Terms like maltodextrin are used for regular terms of sugar, with the intention of hiding it. There are literally hundreds of them, maybe thousands. In my estimation, this is criminal behavior. You can still protect yourself by not buying into it, so don't.

Choose something else to feed your family. You'll be much further ahead in the long run. The money it will save you in pharmaceuticals is nothing short of astounding. In my estimation, this is criminal behavior. It's criminal behavior being done on an industrial level. Monsanto has politically engineered their control of the FDA and USDA to ensure their compliance in Monsanto's dominance of our food supply.

That is why I included my third chapter on our celebration of our addiction. Corporate does this on purpose. They do this because they know that we are addicted by our rate of consumption of their wares. They also know that with their lobbying power, they can get away with virtually anything. It's kind of the same situation as that of the military-industrial complex. They support congressmen and senators in every state and district, securing their interests, with this influence. Monsanto has even gone to the extent of contracting every farmer that they can, even to the point of suing farmers, just to corner the market. The last corporations that got away with this kind of behavior were busted up by Teddy Roosevelt in the late 19th century. No industry in our history has had more influence on our health, either as an individual or as a society than this grain and sugar industry has with its addictive food. No industry may be more influential in the countrol of our health. It's created a multi-trillion dollar medical and pharmaceutical industry. The thing that scares them the most is the ketogenic diet as it's the only diet that can save you and the world, from their clutches.

We allow these corporations to addict us, even worse than we've been any time in the history of man, for which we should be ashamed. I would be but I didn't set up the Supreme Court to allow Monsanto to patent life in patenting GMO seeds. This may end up being the bane of mankind, as it is a very deadly path for our food industry to be taking. But then it's only deadly to those who buy into it. That's why I won't.

XI
FAT - YOUR POWER FOOD

The advantages of being thin, far outweigh just looking better. Of course, there's always simple benefits to being thin, such as being able to stand up easier and get out of bed easier. Most everybody wants to be thin simply to look good, but the advantages of being thin, go a lot further than just looking good. Being thin is not only highly beneficial for your looks it's crucial for your health and even more important for your brain's health. Did you know that the fatter you are, the smaller your brain, is? It's true. That is directly from Dr. Perlmutter's book, *Grain Brain.* Conversely, the thinner you are, the bigger your brain, can be, also. Odds are, you didn't know that either.

Obesity is a danger to more than just your body, it's shrinking your brain by eating it up slowly and it's all due to excessive carbohydrate consumption, carbohydrates in the form of cereals, breads, and pastas. But, we're talking about your body, here. According to Dr. Donald W. Miller, Jr., MD, *"Carbohydrates are the primary cause of weight gain, not fats. (Animals raised for food are fattened with carbohydrates.)"* Remember the Iowa Corn Fed Beef Ruse? How many cows, that you know of, graze on ears of corn? Most cattle I see in a field, are eating grass. *"He goes on to say that eating fat is not only healthier than eating carbohydrates, it makes you thinner."* Yes, it's true, eating fat keeps you thin.

Eating Fat Keeps From Being Fat

Studies have shown that getting back to what our original metabolism likes, for a diet, and what our bodies are meant to digest means getting back to a diet higher in fats and lower in carbohydrates.

Low carb diets began emerging in the mid-to-late-2000s. Studies which evaluate low-carbohydrate diets over much longer periods started showing up in the PubMed and PMC files, dating back to the late 40's and early 50's. Some of these controlled studies were as long as two years and survey studies as long as two decades, show that diets high in protein and fat are much more beneficial than a diet high in carbohydrates.

Dr. Atkins was the first to promote a low carbohydrate diet as early as 1958, yet it seems that the carbohydrate addiction complex had already started its devious work in addicting our society to the ravages of the *Wheat Belly* saga. It seems that too many of the USDA and FDA thought it better to restrict our consumption of fats, thinking that's what was causing all the problem with obesity and diabetes. In all actuality, it's carbs that cause the fat that causes obesity and diabetes, not fat at all. It's the process of turning those carbs into fat that's at the foundation of all disease, the action of insulin turning glucose into fat.

A question I have to ask, did Monsanto and their cronies in the USDA and FDA know about this, when these decisions were made? I'm sure Monsanto was aware of what glycation and their glyphosate does for that glycation, as they'd been researching it for years, at that point. If more of this information were more readily available to the public, as it's released, wouldn't that give the public a better opportunity to know and fully appreciate, all the ramifications of this addiction?

Physically, it's all a matter of how they are digested. To digest carbohydrates, your body has to turn them into fat. This is because your body can't run on sugar. It runs on fat. What this means is that when you eat carbohydrates, your body can't use that as food because it burns fat. That's where your insulin comes into play. The problem with that is your insulin also instructs that fat to go to storage, which starts in the visceral fat around the midsection. Eating carbs, demands the insulin, that turns those carbs into visceral fat, except that this visceral fat is barely usable. You can use it, but there are better fuels, to use. And, because this is barely usable and it always comes with a lot more fat with it, it's designated as visceral fat by the body and it attracts more fat to join it. This is the fat that demands more fat to join it, through leptin resistance..

When you eat fat, your body doesn't have to convert that into anything to use. It's digested in your small intestine, unlike carbs that are metabolized cellularly with the help of insulin. That means that the glucose that carbs become, have to float around in your bloodstream until they can enter a cell to be used as glycogen. This is where the problem begins. Anyone who's been on a diet of carbohydrates for any amount of time has trouble making enough insulin to convert the glucose into fat, so it can be used for fuel. The problem with this requirement of getting your fuel in this way is that the insulin needed to turn the carb into fat instructs that fat to go directly to storage (usually because more is on the way). So it goes to visceral fat around the midsection for men and the thighs and hips for women. This is what can't be avoided when eating a carbohydrate diet. Insulin turns the glucose into triglycerides which turn into IDL then VLDL then LDL, but this LDL isn't clean burning LDL. It's contaminated with glyphosated glycation that does nothing but gum up your cells and alter your hormonal health.

The cholesterol this fat makes is ApoB which is the foundation of more disease than any other type of cholesterol. It's a sticky kind of cholesterol and is why it collects as visceral fat around the mid section where it adheres to your organs. It's here that it demands more fat to join it, to start your metabolic syndrome.

The first place your body stores this fat is around your midsection, hence its name, belly fat or visceral fat. This is a dangerous fat to have in your body as this is where diabetes starts, along with a host of cancers and CVDs or heart diseases and most every kind of dementia, including Alzheimer's Disease, Parkinson's Disease, and Huntington's Disease. Human biology hasn't changed, evolutionarily enough, to allow humans to continue to eat carbohydrates in the massive amounts that everyone everywhere is eating them.

The Paleo Diet is a recent addition to the low carb diet choice. The ketogenic diet is the ultimate in a low carb diet and has already shown numerous benefits for better health. It's the recommended diet for Celiac Disease since Celiac Disease is caused by the gluten that's found in wheat, barley and rye and a few other grains. It's also the oldest low carb diet, first designed in 1921, to help control epilepsy and seizures. The diet fell out of use when seizure medicines became more prevalent, (along with the side effects). And, we're not even covering the ecological impact, or environmental impact, or societal impact, with the terrorism, this carbohydrate has diet increased,

It turns out that a ketogenic diet is the healthiest diet that any human can eat. It goes back to the way our bodies have metabolized food for the last 100,000 years. Simply because this diet is based on fat and not carbs, the diet provides much higher octane fuel for our bodies to use. Carbohydrates have a tendency to gum up your body. They do it by creating plaque. That gets into to glycation of proteins and LDL cholesterol, which you've already read about in chapter IV, *The Danger of Glycation.*

This plaque buildup is the foundation of 75% of the deadliest and costliest diseases, known to man, ranging from breast cancer to Atherosclerosis to 95% of all dementias, making carbohydrates some of the deadliest food that any human can eat. It's not, that this food just makes us fat, it kills us slowly, painfully, and expensively, with an arm-long list of disorders. For this one reason alone, the power of being thin, cannot be over spoken.

Studies have also shown the simple practice of calorie restriction to have multiple beneficial effects on the body, least of which is extended life. It's amazing what just going hungry, can do for your body. It ramps up your immune system by boosting your anti-oxidants exponentially. While doing that, it actually helps your brain grow, through a little protein in your brain known as *BDNF,* brain-derived neurotrophic factor. This is what makes your brain grow and it doesn't happen, as much, in obese people. This is part of the power of being thin.

Calorie restriction on a carbohydrate diet is next to impossible, yet I do it every day and quite easily and comfortably, on my MCT ketogenic diet. An MCT ketogenic diet is, in my estimation, the easiest low carbohydrate diet to get adjusted to. MCTs (Medium Chain Triglycerides) work differently in your body than LCTs (Long Chain Triglycerides). MCTs are a good way to actually lower your cholesterol because they build up the HDL cholesterol. Coconut oil is optimal for this, as it contains lauric acid and lauric acid is the foundation of HDL's Apolipoprotein A cholesterol, the good cholesterol.

I'm compelled to agree with what Dr. Miller had included in his paper, *"calorie restriction prolongs life as well as contributes to an increase in mental capabilities."* This is the true power of being thin. It comes easiest from being on a high-fat low carb diet.

The Value of Balancing Your Cholesterol

Too often I hear the phrase I've got to get my cholesterol down. People saying this think that high cholesterol is something to fear. High cholesterol isn't nearly as big of a problem as unbalanced cholesterol. Cholesterol is a very important part of bodily functions and plays a major impact on your health.

To lower one's cholesterol is to endanger one's health.

"Low cholesterol has been connected to depression, anxiety, bipolar disorder and statistically higher frequency of violent behavior, suicide, Parkinson's disease, and cancer mortality. Susceptibilities to tuberculosis and gastrointestinal infections are also associated with lower cholesterol levels. Most significantly, the death rate is doubled in older adults with lower total cholesterol and stroke and cataracts rates are higher." That was according to **The Great Plains Laboratory**, but you can find the same message from multiple sources, proclaiming the dangers of low cholesterol.

Dr. Mercola says;

"The Risks of Low Cholesterol
impaired memory and dementia are just the tip of the iceberg when it comes to low cholesterol's impact on your brain. Having too little of this beneficial compound also:
- *Increases your **risk of depression***
- *Can **cause you to commit suicide***
- *May lead to **violent behavior and aggression***
- *Increase your **risk of cancer** and Parkinson's disease*

"Unfortunately, in the united states lowering cholesterol levels has become so common that nearly everyone reading this either knows someone struggling to do so, or has struggled to do so themselves." Why is our medical industry persuading us to lower cholesterol, when it's so important? Is that because it leads to more medication? Is this an FDA directive? We all know, who controls them.

CHOLESTEROL IS NOT THE ENEMY

"Since cholesterol is essential for all animal life, each cell synthesizes it through a complex process beginning with the mevalonate pathway and ending with a 19 step conversion of lanosterol to cholesterol. Increased dietary intake of industrial trans fats, but not ruminant saturated fats(including cholesterol), is associated with an increased risk in all-cause mortality, cardiovascular diseases or type 2 diabetes."
"Most ingested cholesterol is esterified, and esterified cholesterol is poorly absorbed. The body also compensates for any absorption of additional cholesterol by reducing cholesterol synthesis " "Biosynthesis of cholesterol is directly regulated by the cholesterol levels present, though
the homeostatic mechanisms involved are only partly understood. A higher intake from food leads to a net decrease in endogenous production, whereas lower intake from food has the opposite effect." Simply stated, the more you eat, the less you make. But because most ingested cholesterol is esterified, it's important to know where these fats come from.
"In addition to its importance within cells, cholesterol also serves as a precursor for the biosynthesis of steroid hormones, bile acids, and vitamin D"

Cholesterol is crucial in the manufacture of hormones for the body's function. As vitamin D is crucial for brain function, cholesterol is crucial in the manufacture of vitamin D. This is why statin drugs that are made for lowering cholesterol, are so dangerous.

With a substance as vital as this seems to appear, why do people want to lower it? Maybe we should look at how it's transported to your cells and what role that plays in the cholesterol equation.

Cholesterol is transported inside **lipoproteins**.

Cholesterol comes in many forms of lipoproteins, HDL (High-Density Lipoproteins), LDL (Low-Density Lipoproteins), and VLDL (Very Low-Density Lipoproteins) just to name a few. This is where is gets interesting,

According to Wikipedia;
"Low-density lipoprotein (LDL) is one of the five major groups of lipoproteins. These groups, from least dense to most dense, are chylomicrons, very low-density lipoprotein (VLDL), intermediate-density lipoprotein (IDL), low-density lipoprotein and high-density lipoprotein (HDL), all of them, particles far smaller than human cells. In nutrition, LDL is sometimes referred to as the "bad cholesterol".

"Lipoproteins transfer fats around the body in the extracellular fluid can be sampled from blood and allow fats to be taken up by the cells of the body by receptor-mediated endocytosis. Lipoproteins are complex particles composed of multiple proteins which transport all fat molecules (lipids) around the body within the water outside cells. They are typically composed of 80-100 proteins/particle (organized by a single apolipoprotein B for LDL and the larger particles). A single LDL particle is about 260-300 nm in diameter (submicroscopic) typically transporting 3,000 to 6,000 fat molecules/particle, varying in size according to the number and mix of fat molecules contained within. The fats carried include cholesterol, phospholipids, and triglycerides; amounts of each vary considerably."

"LDL particles vary in size and density, and studies have shown that a pattern that has more small dense LDL particles, called Pattern B, *equates to a higher risk factor for coronary heart disease (CHD) than does a pattern with more of the larger and less-dense LDL particles (Pattern A)."*

*"LDL particles pose a risk for **cardiovascular disease** when they invade the **endothelium** and become **oxidized** since the oxidized forms are more easily retained by the proteoglycans. A complex set of biochemical reactions regulates the oxidation of LDL particles, chiefly stimulated by the presence of necrotic cell debris and **free radicals** in the endothelium. Increasing concentrations of LDL particles are strongly associated with increasing rates of accumulation of **atherosclerosis** within the walls of arteries over time, eventually resulting in **sudden plaque ruptures** and triggering clots within the artery opening, or a narrowing or closing of the opening, I.E. cardiovascular disease, **stroke**, and other **vascular disease** complications."*

It's easy to see now, the importance of lowering ApoB LDL. This is what The National Library of medicine has to say about **cholesterol ratios;**

"Low-density lipoprotein (LDL) cholesterol concentration has been the prime index of cardiovascular disease risk and the main target for therapy. However, several lipoprotein ratios or "atherogenic indices" have been defined in an attempt to optimize the predictive capacity of the lipid profile. In this review, we summarize their pathophysiological aspects and highlight the rationale for using these lipoprotein ratios as cardiovascular risk factors in clinical practice, specifying their cut-off risk levels and a target for lipid-lowering therapy. Total/high-density lipoprotein (HDL) cholesterol and LDL/HDL cholesterol ratios are risk indicators with greater predictive value than isolated parameters used independently, particularly LDL. Future recommendations regarding the diagnosis and treatment of dyslipidemia, including instruments for calculating cardiovascular risk or action guidelines, should include the lipoprotein ratios with the greater predictive power which, in view of the evidence-based results, are none other than those which include HDL cholesterol." With the advantages of HDL as opposed to the disadvantages of LDL, it's become important to know the difference in HDL and LDL because a balance in the ratio seems to be more important than anything else.

This is why HDL particles are so important. This is because these particles are considered cell scrubbers, because they clean out your spent LDL after the cell burns it. If that can't get cleaned out of your cells, the LDL backs up in your blood, and waits to be glycated.
That says to me, what's important to know is how to create HDL and how to not create LDL. This will go much farther than any medicine to balance HDL/LDL cholesterol.

Wikipedia goes on to say;

*"**HDL particles** remove fats and cholesterol from cells, including within **artery** wall **atheroma**, and transport it back to the liver for excretion or re-utilization; thus the cholesterol carried within HDL particles (HDL-C) is sometimes called "good cholesterol" (despite being the same as cholesterol in LDL particles)."*
*"Increasing concentrations of HDL particles are strongly associated with decreasing accumulation of atherosclerosis within the walls of arteries. This is important because atherosclerosis eventually results in **sudden plaque ruptures, cardiovascular disease, stroke** and other **vascular diseases**. HDL particles are sometimes referred to as "good cholesterol" because they can transport fat molecules out of*

artery walls, reduce macrophage accumulation, and thus help prevent or even regress atherosclerosis."
"High LDL with low HDL level is an additional risk factor for cardiovascular disease. ·· In a large sample of middle-aged adults, low HDL cholesterol was associated with poor memory and decreasing levels over a five-year follow-up period were associated with a decline in memory

Low HDL, low memory. That's interesting, with all that said from Wikipedia, it's easy to see that not all cholesterol is equal. Some are good and some are bad. Thus, the "good cholesterol, bad cholesterol mantra", which more than anything boasts the value of balancing your cholesterol, rather than lowering it. The paragraph above about HDL cholesterol says it all, increasing HDL cholesterol is a good thing, as it's *"associated with decreasing accumulation of atherosclerosis within the cell walls of the arteries".*

As you can see, HDL, the good cholesterol is something you want in your body, but the LDL, bad cholesterol is something to regulate levels in your body. And, you can do this with what you eat, as that dictates what apolipoprotein will be at the core of the cholesterol, which dictates which kind of particle it'll go into, LDL or HDL. Wikipedia goes on to say about HDL;

"HDL is the smallest of the lipoprotein particles. It is the densest because it contains the highest proportion of protein to lipids. Its most abundant apolipoproteins are apo A-I and apo A-II. (A rare genetic variant, ApoA-1 Milano, has been documented to be far more effective in both protecting against and regressing arterial disease; atherosclerosis). The liver synthesizes these lipoproteins as complexes of apolipoproteins and phospholipid, which resemble cholesterol-free flattened spherical lipoprotein particles; the complexes are capable of picking up cholesterol, carried internally, from cells by interaction with the ATP-binding cassette transporter A1 (ABCA1). A plasma enzyme called lecithin-cholesterol acyltransferase (LCAT) converts the free cholesterol into cholesteryl ester (a more hydrophobic form of cholesterol), which is then sequestered into the core of the lipoprotein particle, eventually causing the newly synthesized HDL to assume a spherical shape. HDL particles increase in size as they circulate through the bloodstream and incorporate

more cholesterol and phospholipid molecules from cells and other lipoproteins, for example by the interaction with the ABCG1 transporter and the phospholipid transport protein (PLTP)."

*"HDL transports cholesterol mostly to the **liver** or **steroidogenic organs** such as **adrenals**, **ovary**, and **testes** by both direct and indirect pathways. HDL is removed by HDL receptors such as **scavenger receptor BI** (SR-BI), which mediate the selective uptake of cholesterol from HDL. In humans, probably the most relevant pathway is the indirect one, which is mediated by **cholesteryl ester transfer protein (CETP)**. This protein exchanges triglycerides of **VLDL** against cholesteryl esters of HDL. As the result, VLDLs are processed to **LDL**, which are removed from the circulation by the **LDL receptor** pathway. The triglycerides are not stable in HDL, but are degraded by **hepatic lipase** so that, finally, small HDL particles are left, which restart the uptake of cholesterol from cells."*

"The cholesterol delivered to the liver is excreted into the **bile** and, hence, **intestine** either directly or indirectly after conversion into **bile acids**. Delivery of HDL cholesterol to adrenals, ovaries, and testes is important for the synthesis of **steroid hormones**."

This is why it's important to get all your cholesterol into high-density lipoproteins to transfer fats from cells, where they can be used to do the most good. Eating MCT's are the quickest to build up your HDL particles. With more HDL particles to clean the LDL out of the cells, your LDL particles automatically decrease, balancing your cholesterol instead of just lowering it. Why zap your energy, when you don't have to.

It seems the loose floating fats, the triglycerides, VLDL and LDL cholesterol are more open, for glycation by loose glucose in the system than the tighter more compact fats contained in the HDL packets, making them more likely to become glycated and turned into plaque. Since it's the carbohydrates that contribute most to your triglycerides, curbing your carbs goes furthest in limiting your triglycerides.

All the evidence show that eating fat raises HDL. As long as it's healthy saturated fats, MTC fats. Wow! Eating fat increases my HDL and lowers my LDL? *"What a Deal!"* It does that by balancing the ratio. That's what's important. As long as the cholesterol is moving through the cells, and moving freely (which means that it has to be clean). That means that your cholesterol shouldn't come from carbs, to stay clean. Clean cholesterol, HDL raising cholesterol comes from fat, saturated fat. Sound like a myth? It's the stone cold truth, as proven by the reports.

But you'll find that your total over-all cholesterol will improve your health and increase your energy, exponentially. This is another myth of the carb industry. This proves how healthy, eating fat is. With that said, balancing your cholesterol seems to be much more important than just lowering your cholesterol. You really don't want to lower your good cholesterol, the HDL, because of all the good it does, yet, instead of lowering, balancing the LDL with all the damage that can do, would be wise. So what is a good way to balance your cholesterol?

There are several ways;

1. *"Certain changes in diet and exercise may have a positive impact on raising HDL levels:*
2. *Decreased intake of simple carbohydrates.*
3. *Aerobic exercise,*
4. *Weight loss,*
5. *Magnesium supplements raise HDL-C.*
6. *Addition of soluble fiber to diet (Curb the starchy carbs and trade them for fruits and vegetables)*
7. *Consumption of omega-3 fatty acids such as fish oil or flax oil*
8. *Consumption of medium-chain triglycerides (MCTs) such as caproic acid, caprylic acid, capric acid, and lauric acid.*
9. *Removal of trans fatty acids from the diet*
10. *Most saturated fats increase HDL cholesterol to varying degrees and also raise total and LDL cholesterol. A high-fat, adequate-protein, low-carbohydrate ketogenic diet may have a similar response to taking niacin (vitamin B3) through beta-hydroxybutyrate coupling the Niacin receptor 1.*

- **MCTs from coconut oil increase HDL cholesterol.**

"MCTs passively diffuse from the GI tract to the portal system without the requirement for modification of long-chain fatty acids or very-long-chain fatty acids(longer fatty acids are absorbed into the lymphatic system). In addition, MCTs do not require bile salts for digestion. Patients who have malnutrition, malabsorption or particular fatty-acid metabolism disorders are treated with MCTs because MCTs do not require energy for absorption, use, or storage."

"Some studies have shown that MCTs can help in the process of excess calorie burning, thus weight loss. MCTs are also seen as promoting fat oxidation and reduced food intake."

Medium Chain Triglycerides come from Coconut oil, Palm Kernel oil, and dairy fats. That means that butter and cheese can actually help you lose weight and balance your cholesterol. How great is that? You can go back to eating butter with healthier consequences than eating margarine.

"Coconut milk is rich in medium-chain fatty acids (MCFAs), which the body processes differently from other saturated fats. If MCFAs are used in a diet to replace long-chain fatty acids (LCFAs) such as animal fats they may help promote weight maintenance without raising cholesterol levels.

"Coconut milk contains a large proportion of lauric acid, a saturated fat that raises blood cholesterol levels by increasing the amount of high-density lipoprotein cholesterol" Like coconut oil and milk, bovine milk is high in Lauric Acid.

"Medium-chain triglycerides are generally considered a good biologically inert source of energy that the human body finds reasonably easy to metabolize. They have potentially beneficial attributes in protein metabolism but may be contraindicated in some situations due to a reported tendency to induce ketogenesis and metabolic acidosis. However, there is another authority reporting no risk of ketoacidosis or ketonemia with MCTs at levels associated with normal consumption."

"Due to their ability to be absorbed rapidly by the body, medium-chain triglycerides have found use in the treatment of a variety of malabsorption ailments. MCT supplementation with a low-fat diet has been described as the cornerstone of treatment for Waldmann disease. MCTs are an ingredient in some specialized parenteral nutritional emulsions in some countries (not the USA). Studies have also shown promising results for neurodegenerative disorders (e.g. Alzheimer's and

Parkinson's diseases) and epilepsy through the use of ketogenic dieting.
"MCFA (chain lengths of 10 carbons or less are found in greatest concentrations in coconut oil, approximately 14% by weight but can also be found in butter (approximately 9.2%) and palm kernel oil (approximately 7.2%)" "MCT oil has been taunted as a potential weight-lowering agent."
According to the US National Library of Science, The *"Weight-loss diet that includes consumption of medium-chain triacylglycerol oil leads to a greater rate of weight and fat mass loss than does olive oil"*
"Thirty-one subjects completed the study (body mass index: 29.8 ± 0.4, in kg/m^2). MCT oil consumption resulted in lower endpoint body weight than did olive oil (−1.67 ± 0.67 kg, unadjusted P = 0.013). There was a trend toward greater loss of fat mass (P = 0.071) and trunk fat mass (P = 0.10) with MCT consumption than with olive oil. Endpoint trunk fat mass, total fat mass, and intra-abdominal adipose tissue were all lower with MCT consumption than with olive oil consumption (all unadjusted P values < 0.05)."

In my attempt to find what fats create ApoB LDL, I've found one reference that saturated fat contributes to the formation of LDL. Yet, I've also found plenty of **data** that suggests, where the bulk of this kind of cholesterol comes from. All that I've researched shows that ApoB cholesterol comes from glucose. Glucose that comes from starchy carbohydrates. It all has to do with the digestion of carbs. These fats are apportioned to the visceral fat around the belly instead of fats you can use for immediate fuel and this is where it's formed into LDL, most often with Apo B at its core, with the help of Ribosomes from your liver. This is also where it becomes so dangerous.

Again, according to Wikipedia, *"Lowering the blood lipid concentration of triglycerides helps lower the concentration of small LDL particles because fatty-acid rich VLDL particles convert in the bloodstream into small dense LDL particles."*

It makes sense then, if you want to stop the productions of ApoB LDL, you need to stop the production of triglycerides, the fuel that feeds the worst of it, and the best way to stop that, is to curb the high starchy carbohydrates from the worst offenders, grain-based foods. The guiltiest of the group is wheat, followed closely by soy, corn, then rice and oats. All grain-based foods are at the top of this list, along with starchy vegetables like potatoes, parsnips, and carrots, although carrots do have some nutritional value, like beta-carotene. All the others just don't carry enough nutrition to counterbalance the load of carbs you get, with them.

If you're not ready to give up your carbs, there are alternatives, to help you lower your LDL, *"Niacin (B3), lowers LDL by selectively inhibiting hepatic diacylglycerol acyltransferase 2, reducing triglyceride synthesis and VLDL secretion through a receptor HM74 and HM74A or GPR109A" "A ketogenic diet may have similar response to taking niacin (lowered LDL and increased HDL) through beta-hydroxybutyrate, a ketone body, coupling the niacin receptor (HM74A)."*

Statin drugs are made to lower LDL also, but I can only recommend steering clear of those, as they cause too many problems in their action of lowering LDL. As a certified caregiver, I've seen, too often, the ravages this drug commits the body to. They are nothing short of devastating. In every case of a patient I took care of, the patient died prematurely from the side effects of these drugs. It seems to me that in our attempt to cure ourselves, we're killing ourselves. Cholesterol is just too important to lower.

So, an MCT ketogenic diet can not only help you balance your cholesterol but it can help you lose weight and keep it off forever Who knew that coconut oil or coconut milk could be so healthy? Who knew that butter could be so healthy? I certainly didn't, but I do now. Who knew that whole milk is ten times healthier than low-fat or nonfat milk? Who knew, that whole milks are not dangerous, in the least? Because of its cholesterol balancing properties, they're, really very healthy. Has your doctor ever shared this information with you? Does this information carry with it the need for further care? Maybe, that's why.

Because MCT ketogenic diets are made for calorie restriction and this next point deals with calorie restriction, I can see the benefits here, as well, for added **BDNF for brain growth, increased Nrf2 for anti-oxidant production.**

FIND YOUR CURE

THAT YOU KNOW IS PURE

AND LASTS FOREVER THAT'S FOR SURE

BUT, YOU MUST IGNORE THE LURE

TO NOT EAT WHAT IS COMPLETELY IMPURE

WHICH INCLUDES ALL GRAINS, AND THAT'S FOR SURE

IT'S UP TO YOU TO AVOID THIS RUSE

AND PAY THE DUES YOU'LL FOREVER RUE

AS ONLY YOU WILL FEEL ITS BLUES

FASTING BRINGS RETURN TO HEALTH

THAT HELPS YOU KEEP

YOUR WELL EARNED WEALTH

WITHOUT THE NEED FOR MEDICATION

IT GETS RETURNED

BY HORMONE DESTAGNATION

TO BRING BACK A LIBERATION

FROM YOUR ONGOING,

STAGNATING, GLYCATION

XII

The Bliss of Ketosis.

I can remember growing up as a toddler, my father had an answer for everything I asked. That lasted, until I turned 30. That was the year my life changed. And, it wasn't really to my liking. Actually, it was by far, the most detrimental thing that could happen to anyone. That's the question my dad couldn't answer, "why'd this happen to me?"

Mom, on the other hand, answered all my questions until I was probably a senior in high-school when I'd get an answer like "you'd have to ask your dad. I don't know". Both of my parents were smart, but uneducated beyond high-school. My father had this insatiable appetite to better his brain, I think in an attempt to forestall the damaging of his. Mom, on the other hand, was content do what she could to just keep up.

Mom loved bread. I think that's why she could only do her best to "just keep up" with raising 3 kids after her first two children died 1 and 2 days after childbirth. Those were my twin brothers, Ronald and Roger. All my life, I've visited their graves, with Mom and Dad in the Wayne cemetery, the town I remember living in from 8 months old to 8 years old. It's where all of our remains will be buried, as I'm their only surviving son.

I've not done too much, that I'm proud of. On the other hand, I've done far too much that I'm ashamed of, like not getting an education, like treating people in ways that I know I shouldn't and taking ill-advised chances that were unnecessary. My sins are many and I wish like hell, I had used better sense, before I acted those ill times that I did. I wish now that I could've had enough sense to consider the consequences of my actions, like my parents had taught me, prior to my acting like I did and doing what I did.

It really was too bad that I had better notions, that I thought I knew better. I wish now, that I had listened to Mom & Dad when they told me to think before acting, because it's that lack of thinking that created so much turmoil throughout my entire life, culminating with a severe closed head injury that forever changed what goals I ever had for my life. This, combined with all of my subsequent injuries have given me several reasons to look back and reflect, what if I had thought first?

Would I change things, if I could? You bet. I believe anyone who says that they'd never change anything, hasn't learned anything. Either that, or they're happy with the lesson they learned from those errors, and wouldn't have preferred to learn other lessons.

Me? I'd change just about everything I ever did, due to the fact that most of what I've accomplished was tainted with wrong motives or ill-advised actions, producing questionable results that could have been avoided if I had only thought first. I would happily exhange my lessons for other lessons that wouldn't have hurt so many other people.

Unfortunately, I was always in too big of a hurry to work carefully or thoughtfully. This was due to two things;
1. Excess sugar consumption mostly in the form of PB&J sandwiches, the unbounded supply of snacks and cookies (my mother loved to bake from all the smiles it put on me and my sister's faces). I have fond memories of eating *Sugar Pops, Cocoa Puffs,* and loving them, terribly. This created an insatiable hunger in me to accomplish my tasks quickly, often instantly, because I didn't want to wait for results.
2. My lack of education. This didn't allow me to take the time I needed to assess, research and examine my situations and options prior to my acting which, ultimately, set me up to lose dramatically all that I had gained in my life up to that point.

Even though I did complete two years of college and graduated with an A.A. degree, my grade point average was so low, with the exception of Music Theory, beyond my 1st year, I learned virtually nothing. This was due to various learning disabilities combined with unexpected occurrences that life has a habit of bringing about. The learning disabilities? I didn't know, at the time that I had them.

I didn't learn, until recently that I have ADD, and may have suffered with ADHD when I was in school. It's hard to say what the underlying factors were, but my second year in college was pretty much a waste of time and money, for which I'll forever regret.

My learning disabilities were all initiated by my consumption of those cookies that Mom was always making for me. And, I loved to eat them, plenty of them. And, the sugar proceeded to do its damage. Too bad Mom didn't know that my runny nose only matched my running feet because of the excess sugar consumption. I wish that she had known that even just a little sugar, can be as deadly as a little arsenic. The sugar just kills slower. That's because it's gummier and gluier than the arsenic is, making it a slower murderer.

Armed with this information, I choose to remain on my ketogenic diet of bacon and milk. Actually, I include yogurt, cheese, eggs, and other meats for sources of protein, with raw nuts and some seeds, like pumpkin.

This is where carboholics do not have the advantage that I and other ketonemiacs have. Ketonemiacs aren't controlled by their hormones, so we don't have to follow any hunger cycle. We're in full control of our hormones. This also means that we're in more control of our emotions because of that. I know that it doesn't sound like it's that big of a deal, but it's more important than you could ever, imagine. Whether you want to call me a ketonemaic or a ketomaniac, either is fine with me. Ketomania has gained full control of my body.

The biggest confusion with being in a state of ketosis is that it is often confused with ketoacidosis, which has nothing to do with being in a state of nutritional ketosis. Ketoacidosis is a state of extreme ketosis that can only happen to type 1 diabetics because their pancreas is incapable of secreting enough insulin to handle even a small amount of glucose in the system. Because of this the liver of type 1 diabetics secrete more ketones than what the body needs to operate. First, let's look at the state of ketosis, as explained in Wikipedia;

"Ketosis is a metabolic state in which most of the body's energy supply comes from ketone bodies in the blood, in contrast to a state of glycolysis in which blood glucose provides most of the energy.

Ketosis is similar to a condition called **KETOACIDOSIS**, *in that both cause a side effect known to laypeople as acetone breath."*
"Longer-term ketosis may result from fasting or staying on a low-carbohydrate diet, and deliberately induced ketosis serves as a medical intervention for various conditions, such as intractable epilepsy, and the various types of diabetes. In glycolysis, higher levels of insulin promote storage of body fat and block the release of fat from adipose tissues, while in ketosis, fat reserves are readily released and consumed. For this reason, ketosis is sometimes referred to as the body's "fat burning" mode."

Even bodybuilders have recognized ketonemia as being the most beneficial state to keep their body in, as it's in this state, where they produce more growth hormones because of the amount of Ghrelin their stomachs release to enable them to grow their muscles bigger without the carbs. Remember the study that showed the accumulation of HDL cholesterol is used to build hormonal steroids? That comes from a ketogenic diet.

*"Ketosis is deliberately induced by use of a **ketogenic diet** as a medical intervention in cases of intractable **epilepsy**. Other uses of **low-carbohydrate diets** remain controversial. Induced ketosis or low-carbohydrate diet terms have very wide interpretation. Therefore, Stephen S. Phinney and Jeff S. Volek coined the term "nutritional ketosis" to avoid the confusion."*

Although I appreciate ketosis as being a "fat burning mode", it's the other benefits that I appreciate more. Benefits like less pain, no headaches, no stomachaches, far more energy than what I've ever had, ability to get more work done, as I don't have to stop all the time to eat and although I do eat at my desk, I'm usually at my desk 16-18 hours out of the day, except on therapy days. I take 3 hours, 3 days a week for therapy. My therapy is exercise. My brain needs it, but my body benefits.

Ketoacidosis is a state of extreme ketosis that can only happen to type 1 diabetics because their pancreas is incapable of secreting enough insulin to handle a large amount of glucose in the system. This is a product of over eating carbohydrates. Because of this, the liver of type 1 diabetics secrete more ketones than what the body needs to operate. this can only happen if you dump excess carbs into your body, either through over eating of over drinking alcohol. (This can't happen to anyone on a ketogenic diet.) Again Wikipedia says on the subject of ketosis;

"Ketoacidosis is a metabolic state associated with high concentrations of ketone bodies, formed by the breakdown of fatty acids and the deamination of amino acids. Ketoacidosis is most common in untreated type 1 diabetes mellitus when the liver breaks down fat and proteins in response to a perceived need for a respiratory substrate. Prolonged alcoholism may lead to alcoholic ketoacidosis."

"In diabetic ketoacidosis, a high concentration of ketone bodies is usually accompanied by insulin deficiency, hyperglycemia, and dehydration. Particularly in type 1 diabetics the lack of insulin in the bloodstream prevents glucose absorption, thereby inhibiting the production of oxaloacetate (a crucial precursor to the β-oxidation of fatty acids) through reduced levels of pyruvate (a byproduct of glycolysis), and can cause unchecked ketone body production (through fatty acid metabolism) potentially leading to dangerous glucose and ketone levels in the blood. Hyperglycemia results in glucose overloading the kidneys and spilling into the urine (transport maximum for glucose is exceeded). Dehydration results following the osmotic movement of water into urine. (Osmotic diuresis), exacerbates the acidosis."

"I bring this up to make the point that nutritional ketosis is not ketoacidosis. It's far from it. According to Wikipedia again,

"Normal serum reference ranges for ketone bodies are 0.5–3.0 mg/dL, equivalent to 0.05–0.29 mmol/L.[23]" In ketosis, the levels range from 3 – 6 mg/dL. Ketoacidosis requires a level of 15 25 mg/dL, more the three times needed for ketosis, making it virtually impossible for anyone to into ketoacidosis if you're not a type 1 diabetic. Type 1 diabetics are required to make sure their bodies don't produce many ketones because of the risk of ketoacidosis".

Ketoacidosis can only happen by putting carbs in your body. If no carbs go in, ketoacidosis can't possibly happen. Has your doctor shared that with you? Remaining in a state of ketosis, on the other hand, has allowed my body to regain that which was lost 31 years ago in a car accident that left me severely disabled because of a severe closed head injury, (It was the two strokes that were the most devastating.)

Probably the first and foremost reason I choose to remain on this diet is explained by my lack of need for any of these diabetes medications;

1. *insulin*
2. *exenatide*
3. *liraglutide*
4. *pramlintide*
5. *Biguanides*
6. *metformin*
7. **Phenformin**- **Phenformin** *(DBI) was used from the 1960s through 1980s but was withdrawn due to lactic acidosis risk.*
8. **Buformin** - *also was withdrawn due to lactic acidosis risk.*
9. *Thiazolidinediones;*
10. *Rosiglitazone - (Avandia): the* **European Medicines Agency** *recommended in September 2010 that it be suspended from the EU market due to elevated cardiovascular risks.*
11. *Pioglitazone*
12. **Troglitazone** *- (Rezulin): used in the 1990s, withdrawn due to* **hepatitis** *and liver damage risk*
13. Peptide analogs;
14. **Secretagogues***;   First-generation agents*
15. *tolbutamide*
16. *acetohexamide*
17. *tolazamide*
18. *chlorpropamide*
19. Second-generation agents;
20. *glipizide*
21. *glyburide or* **glibenclamide**
22. *glimepiride*
23. *gliclazide*
24. *gliquidone*
25. *Meglitinides*
26. *repaglinide*
27. *nateglinide*
28. *Alpha-glucosidase inhibitors*
29. *miglitol*
30. *acarbose*
31. *voglibose*
32. Injectable Amylin analogs
33. *Amylin*
34. *pramlintide*
35. *SGLT-2 inhibitors*

Common generic names for many of these medicines are from Wikipedia; Many anti-diabetes drugs are available as generics. These include;

36. **Sulfonylureas**- *glimepiride, glipizide, glyburide*
37. **Biguanides**- *metformin*
38. **Thiazolidinediones(Tzd)** - *pioglitazone, Actos generic*
39. **Alpha-glucosidase inhibitors**- *Acarbose*
40. **Meglitinides**- *nateglinide*
41. **Combination of sulfonylureas plus metformin** - *known by generic names of the two drugs*

"No generics are available for dipeptidyl peptidase-4 inhibitors (Januvia, Onglyza) and other combinations."

The above medications are used for diabetes alone. This small list is quite possibly the smallest list that one will need to choose from with a continued diet of carbohydrates. Larger lists exist for heart disease, cancer, high blood pressure, high cholesterol, arthritis, and dementia. That only covers the prescription medication. For OCD medication, you have to consider NSAIDs, the most used pain relievers all carrying more side effects to create more need for further medication. And don't forget Tylenol. How many problems does that drug have with liver toxicity? It's been responsible for a few deaths. Then we have to look at the Antacids and all the stomach medicine that's on the shelf. There are plenty of them and I can honestly tell you right now that 90% of these medications are not necessary unless you're on a carbohydrate diet. I haven't used any of these medications in 5 years since I completely gave up the bread and carbs. I still have two or three volumes of drug books full of pharmaceuticals that are needed to treat any of the diseases that are caused by the consumption of grains. They all collect dust.

I refuse to take any of these drugs anymore because all of them carry side effects, some major, some minor. Whether the side effects are major or minor, I don't want to experience any of them. I've had my fill of side effects, especially the ones that make my health worse, which is where most of these side effects should be classified. After living for twenty years needing to take, massive amounts of opioids for my chronic severe pain, along with muscle relaxants, and diuretics for my high blood pressure, anti-depressants for the pain, and living with the side effects of not only the opioids but every other drug they had me on, all twelve of them. I got fed up with it. I wasn't going to take it anymore, and I'm not going to take it anymore, from now on. I was only up to twelve medications. I have a friend who's on this diet, who's lowered his needs to thirteen daily medications from twenty-three. How many meds do you take every day? How many of their side effects would you rather live without?

I live by the theory that if the meds aren't needed in the first place, my health is going to be that much better. That is why I removed everything from my diet that I could, that is responsible for these horrendous diseases, requiring the need for these medications. The one thread I found that ties 80% of all cancers (even lung cancer), 90% of all heart diseases, and 99.9 % of all dementia, all arthritis, all headaches, and almost all stomachaches together is one substance that can be removed from the diet without any severe side effects. I shouldn't need to tell you what that substance is by now. You should know. You eat it every day. You live with the effects of addiction. Pain always comes with addiction.

You eat it every morning, either in your coffee as creamer, with your coffee, as Danish, or in the toast you have, or the cereal you consume. You have it every lunch with your sandwich or burrito and with every dinner with your pasta. I have known several families that would just put a plate of bread on the table every evening. This is the display of addiction, a full out need to satisfy the taste buds by dumping more and more sugar in the body, usually in the form of starchy carbs. (Did I mention the empty beer cans in their garbage?)

The sad part of this whole argument is that I've only covered drugs for diabetes so far. I haven't even touched on drugs for heart disease, cancer, arthritis, high blood pressure, high cholesterol (with statins probably the most dangerous), chronic pain (opioids), fibromyalgia, lupus, Alzheimer's disease, Parkinson's etc, etc. How many side effects do think all these drugs can cause? How many more avenues can this create to develop new drugs to spring upon a mindless public, all clamoring for the newest relief from their pain?

I chose to leave you with this image of drug addiction, because it's all of the consumption of the grain industry's products, that's driving the pharmaceutical industry today, tomorrow, next year, and for the next 500 and beyond. If we don't put an end to this now, our society is doomed to suffer the consequences of their carbohydrate addiction, a diet they're not responsible for. The greed of the grain industry combined with the ambition of the pharmaceutical industry has made us all carboholic slaves to the desires these industries. For me, it's scary how much power we've given these to industries, simply because we listen to their advertising. Those who listen to their advertising, and are influenced by it, fall prey to that influence and become their slaves for life or until they quit consuming the grains. There's very little, difference, than that of alcoholism as the alcoholism is just carbolism magnified, exponentially. That's because alcohol is basically, concentrated sugars.

Anyone who can't control their emotions entirely by themselves, is a slave to their own hormones. Every carboholic is a slave to their emotions and therefore a slave to these industries. The emotions I'm speaking about here are hunger and satiety. You may not classify these emotions, but I submit that they actually are. Satiety is defined as the state of being satisfied. If that is not an emotion, as it expresses feelings of calmness and security, I don't know what is. Hunger, on the other hand, is defined as a strong desire. Is not that an emotion? These emotions are control by both Leptin and Ghrelin, which in turn are controlled by the grain industry, more than anything else.

With emotions being controlled by our hormonal balance like this, how could the influence of anything that modifies that balance, not have an effect on our behavior? It has to. When you combine the drive of an addiction (which is what we're talking about) with the advertisements promoting that addiction, how can it not have an effect on our health and ultimately our society? That is why I make the statement that this cycle has to change. If it doesn't cease, our health as a society will never get better.

Let's go back to addiction, though, for I'm sure you don't consider this an addiction. I understand few caught in an addiction can recognize that addiction when they're feeding it because the addiction has ways of hiding it. You can ask anyone who has to have at least one beer a day. They're not addicted to their beer, as far as they're concerned, yet they have to have it. And often they don't even drink more than just one. But they still have to have that one. That is what makes it an addiction. The body can and does live much better without beer, so it's not a substance the body requires to survive. Yet the beer drinker needs that daily beer to satisfy their addiction. To go without, many times causes more problems because of the work your hormones are doing on your emotions and worse yet your actions by controlling how receptors work in your brain. That makes it a natural thing that you need to do, and not an addiction, to appease that desire to drink the beer. This is the physical manifestation of unwanted hormone change, that this addiction brings, in both alcohol and glucose This is how addiction works and it happens to carboholics too. I know I am a carboholic. The desire for sweets is still with me. It's the last refuge of my addiction. It's something that I get to fight, for the rest of my life. I thank God that the further I get from the day I quit, the easier it gets. Now my wrestling happens in an instant. That's how long it takes to remember mosquito bites.

When I think about this I get angry, for I never asked for this nor could I ever wish for it, or wish it upon anyone else. Yet, there is an industry that is committed to not only continuing this pattern, their goal, is to increase its scope. You can see this in all the advertising. What do you think they're advertising when they show you feel good commercials for their soft drinks, fruit drinks, energy drinks, power bars, cereals, bread, pasta, pastries, candy, etc, etc? They're using your emotions to control your behavior. That's because they can. They already control your hormones and it's your hormones that control your emotions. Is it any wonder that so many are addicted?

In my estimation, this is criminal behavior. It's criminal behavior being done on an industrial level. That is the reason for chapter 3, the celebration of addiction. They do this because they know that we are addicted, by our rate of consumption, of their goodies. They also know that with their lobbying power, they can get away with virtually anything. It's kind of the same situation as that of the military-industrial complex. They support congressmen and senators in every state and district, securing their interests, with this influence.

And we allow it to happen, for which we should be ashamed. I am and I'm doing something about it. I'm pleading with you to do something about it, to stifle the destruction that this cycle continues to express on our society. Only U.S. as consumers, can change this equation. For the health of our society, this has become a "must-have", for, if we don't find our cure here, there may not be one.

THIS IS WHAT YOU NEED TO LEARN,
THAT WHAT YOU EAT SHOULD BE TO BURN
FOR FUEL TO FEED YOUR HUNGRY CELLS
FOOD THAT'S CLEAN OF HELTER SKELTER'S, BELLS
THERE IS ONE TRUTH YOU NEED TO SEE
THAT WHAT YOU EAT IS NOT FREE
OF ALL THE PAIN AND MISERY
THAT'S BOUGHT BY YOUR CARBOHYDRATE GLEE
A TRUTH WE NEED TO WAKE UP TO
IS WHAT THESE GRAINS HAVE THE POWER TO DO
TO TEAR ASUNDER THE HOST IT FEEDS
TO BRING DISORDER, PAIN, AND DISEASE.
THE ANGUISH NEVER ENDS UNTIL
THE HOST IS DEAD UNDER THE HILL.
THE ONLY WAY TO BEAT THIS GAME,
REFUSE THE RUSE TO CLAIM YOUR NAME!
IT'S A SIMPLE DECISION TO FORESTALL YOUR PAIN
ALL YOU DO IS GIVE UP THE GRAIN
IT MAY NOT BE EASY ONCE YOU START
BUT YOU'LL REAP REWARDS OF A HEALTHIER HEART
AS IT'S IN THE GRAINS THAT ONLY GLYCATE
THAT'S MAGNIFIED BY GLYPHOSATE
ALL TO PAD THEIR PROFITS WITHOUT REGARD
DO YOU WONDER WHY LIFE'S SO HARD?
THIS BE MY PLEA TO THEE,
TO ALLOW YOURSELF TO LIVE MORE FREELY;
FREE YOURSELF WITH RESIGNATION

OF YOUR OBLIGATION TO THE DEVESTATION OF
ULTRA-GLYPHOSATED RAMPED UP GLYCATION,
TO CEASE THE EATING OF THE GRAINS
FROM THE PLAINS
TO INITIATE THE LIMITATION
OF YOUR ADDICTIVE ADULATION
TO ENCOURAGE THE ELONGATION
OF YOUR DURATION ON THE ROTATION
OF OUR PLANETOID DESTINATION.
SINCE FASTING BRINGS YOUR LASTING HEALTH
THAT HELPS OU KEEP YOUR WELL-EARNED WEALTH

THIS BE MY PLEA FOR THEE;

SET YOUR SELF TRULY FREE

CURB THY CARBS AND BOOST THE FAT

TO FIND OUT WHERE IT'S REALLY AT!

Don't you think it's time for a cure?

I Do!

The Beginning...

www.ingramcontent.com/pod-product-compliance
Lightning Source LLC
Chambersburg PA
CBHW052250220526
45471CB00001B/277